THE AUTHOR

After his first career as an economist and then building Romany caravans in Norfolk, Ernest Roberts took up teaching yoga in London. He developed an original approach to therapy using aspects of yoga practice in conjunction with the twelve Biochemic Tissue Salts. His therapy produced many cures, and led Ernest on to study homœopathy, at first with Thomas Maughan and then at the newly founded College of Homœopathy.

In 1983 Ernest returned to his home town of Manchester and built up a busy homœopathic practice. He founded the North West College of Homœopathy in 1984.

A TEXTBOOK OF THE PRINCIPLES OF HOMŒOPATHIC PRACTICE

by ERNEST M ROBERTS BA. RSHom.

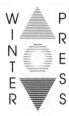

Winter Press
29 Horniman Drive
London SE23 3BJ
First published by Winter Press in 1993

ISBN 1 874581 01 0

Artwork by Neal's Yard DTP Studio, with thanks to their staff
Printed in Great Britain by Biddles of Guildford, Surrey

CONTENTS

LIST OF DIAGRAMS

LIST OF QUOTATIONS

**FROM 'THE ORGANON OF MEDICINE'
BY SAMUEL HAHNEMANN**

Unless otherwise stated all the quotations in the text are from the Organon of Medicine by Samuel Hahnemann, Sixth Edition, in the translation by William Boericke.

Stanza	Page	Stanza	Page
2	2	82	75
3	33, 40, 69	83	51
6	3, 45	143	36
7	37	144	36
9	4	186	27
10	5	187	34
11	21	189	30
12	29	201	32
15	31	210	44
16	21	211	44
18	43	225	33
78	69	226	98

SYMBOLS USED IN THE BOOK
> Symptoms better or ameliorated
< Symptoms worse or aggravated

ACKNOWLEDGEMENTS

I wish to acknowledge the works of George Vithoulkas, Rajan Sankaran and others and thank them for some of the diagrams and ideas I have used from their writings. My thanks to all the help and support from my colleagues who have read, typed and processed the text, and to the students of the North West College of Homœopathy for keeping me ever alert.

This book is dedicated to my son Joseph Carl.

THE PRINCIPLES OF HEALING

An understanding of these twelve principles will provide a clear and firm foundation to Classical Homœopathy. They have been distilled from the Organon and will be explained step by step throughout the following pages.

The page references here refer to the page in this book where you will find the particular principle explained.

PRINCIPLE I

To treat every person as a whole person, not to treat the parts separately but to treat their whole needs. (p2)

PRINCIPLE II

To treat everyone as an individual, to discover what is unique about them and what their whole needs are. (p3)

PRINCIPLE III

To apply a law of minimum interference just sufficient to stimulate the self-healing tendencies in nature and in mankind. We aim to 'restore' not to 'create', to 'destroy' or to 'force'. We work with the forces of the Universe. (p4)

PRINCIPLE IV

The responsibility for our health rests on the choices we make, or fail to make, and what we seek from medical help is advice and guidance as to what these choices are and how to make them. Medical treatment should help us in this process and not seek to help us avoid these choices. (p10)

PRINCIPLE V

There is a natural direction of cure, which is that healing takes place from within outwards, from above downwards, from a vital organ to a less important organ, and in the reverse order of appearance. (p10)

PRINCIPLE VI

Symptoms of disease are desirable manifestations of the body's own intelligent efforts to maintain health. (p20)

PRINCIPLE VII

Health is more dependent on the internal state of our susceptibility than on any external influences. (p20)

PRINCIPLE VIII

Properly conducted provings of single medicinal drugs given to healthy human beings provides Homœopathy with knowledge of the action of the medicines in our Materia Medica. (p35)

PRINCIPLE IX

The principle of using potentised remedies. (p39)

PRINCIPLE X

The principle of similars to enhance patient symptoms in order to strengthen the defensive action of the Vital Force. (p39)

PRINCIPLE XI

The principle of the hierarchical nature of symptoms and its correspondence to the hierarchy found in the natural universe. (p43)

PRINCIPLE XII

Obstacles to cure depend on deep fundamental causes which are accurately described by the Theory of Miasms. These obstacles can be removed by homœopathic treatment. (p78)

FOREWORD

My experiences in teaching homœopathy over the last ten years have convinced me that most of the difficulties encountered in practice arise from a lack of understanding of fundamental principles. Ernest Roberts' book is a welcome treatise that offers a modern step by step guide to unravelling and understanding the apparent complexities of Samuel Hahnemann's masterpiece.

Drawing from both his own experience and a wide range of expert sources such as Kent, Vithoulkas and Sankaran, Ernest Roberts explores various models of health and disease in a clear and extremely readable way. Students and teachers will find this book both thought provoking and a useful reference work.

David Mundy RSHom.

INTRODUCTION

The aim of this book is to help the student to develop a sound understanding of the principles underlying homœopathy. It is intended to be suitable for anyone wishing to learn about the foundations of homœopathy, and as a text-book for students whether at a homœopathic college or medical school, or for those who wish to take up the homœopathic method at any stage of their career.

This book is based on extracts from the founding text of homœopathy, The Organon of Medicine. These extracts are explained in modern terminology, thus helping the student to grasp the principles that will act as their guide when they become homœopathic practitioners.

It is important to begin with The Organon, as this gives us the foundation we call 'Classical'. Only by understanding this foundation can we expect to understand the various schools and methodologies which are advocated throughout the world today by homœopaths. It is my belief that we need to examine the principles underlying each method in order to fully understand it. If the principles that the method is based on are sound, then the therapeutic method may be justifiably employed. So, let us start with the Classical method, and when we have grasped that, we may apply the same rigor to other methods.

Hahnemann's insistence on the empirical foundation of homœopathy and his condemnation of building theories on dogma, belief systems and changing fashions, has led to a rigidity in the minds of some of his followers.

This is particularly true of those who insist only on judging by results, without stating the principles and aims by which to judge these results. Everyone may have good results according to their own criteria, but this begs many questions, such as, what do you mean by a cure?, what is being cured?, what is your hierarchy for grading symptoms? etc.

A second volume will continue and complete the work covered by the Organon and Hahnemann's Chronic Diseases, and then go on to an evaluation and critique of later contributions to homœopathic theory and practice right up to the present day.

Chapter I

A PROFILE OF HEALTH

1.1 INTRODUCTION

In this chapter we will explore what we mean by health and healing. The word 'heal' comes from a root that means to 'make whole'. Hahnemann states that healing the sick is restoring that which has been lost.

> *The highest ideal of cure is rapid, gentle and permanent restoration of the health or removal and annihilation of the disease in its whole extent, in the shortest, most reliable, and most harmless way, on easily comprehensive principles.*
> *(Stanza 2)*

Before we can penetrate how homœopathy works it is necessary to acknowledge that mankind belongs to the Universe or 'one verse' which is beneficent and works for the good of all of its members. This Universe is ruled by natural laws which operate whether or not they are understood correctly or believed in by us. These laws operate in every part of the Universe including the body and psyche of mankind.

To understand the process of healing it is necessary to consider each person as a complete being in the context of their oneness with the Universe and its energy, our first principle of healing is therefore:

PRINCIPLE I

To treat every person as a whole person, not to treat the parts separately but to treat their whole needs.

Stanza 6 of 'The Organon' begins, "The unprejudiced observer..." which refers to the power of observation that Hahnemann constantly urges us to use, and continues "...well aware of the futility of transcendental speculations which can receive no confirmation from experience..." and goes on to assert that the:

*true and only conceivable portrait of the disease is ...only the
deviations from the former healthy state of the now diseased
individual, which are felt by the patient himself, remarked by
those around him and observed by the physician. All these
perceptible signs represent the disease in its whole extent, that
is, together they form the true and only conceivable portrait of
disease.*

(Stanza 6)

Hahnemann is saying here that awareness of healing can only safely be based on observation and understanding of the Laws of Nature as they operate in mankind. For example, the Law of Similars (which is explained in Chapter 2), is like gravity, an empirical law which is observed always to operate. This type of knowledge is known as 'induction'which first observes the facts and then induces laws from these facts. These laws can then be tested in the world by applying them and predicting results which can be seen to be true in life or not. The other approach to knowledge is 'deduction', which takes a set of a-priori postulates from which you deduct by logic certain theories. It is this deductive method that dominates conventional medical thought and produces varied and changing sets of principles according to the variations in the initial premises chosen. Different sets of postulates are chosen by different schools, and postulates are altered as fashions in 'scientific' thinking change. This has led to a medical practice which is a slave to theoretical models and distant from patients' needs.

Also in Stanza 82 we find '... no real cure of ...diseases can take place without a strict particular treatment (individualisation) of each case of disease...' This gives us our second principle of healing:

PRINCIPLE II
To treat everyone as an individual, to discover what is unique about them and what their needs are.

Correct medical healing acknowledges the natural healing forces within each individual which work to repair and restore harmony in the whole being.

> *In the healthy condition of man, the spiritual Vital Force (autocracy), the dynamis that animates the material body (organism), rules with unbounded sway, and retains all the parts of the organism in admirable, harmonious, vital operation, as regards both sensations and functions, so that our indwelling, reason-gifted mind can freely employ this living healthy instrument for the higher purposes of our existence.*
>
> *(Stanza 9)*

The third principle recognises the innate forces that are working towards unity and harmony and that the process of healing seeks to aid them and support them but not to hinder them.

PRINCIPLE III

To apply a law of minimum interference just sufficient to stimulate the self-healing tendencies in nature and in mankind. We aim to 'restore', not to 'force' or to 'destroy'. We work with the natural forces of the Universe.

1.2 MODELS OF MANKIND

There are several models that may be used to help us understand the natural laws and their relationship to man. One model illustrates the different levels of being as a hierarchy:

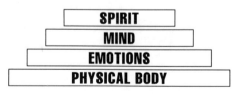

Diagram 1

4

There is a natural hierarchy which pervades the Universe. Equality of honour and the right to be is accorded to every member of each of the four kingdoms; mineral, vegetable, animal and human. However, there is clearly an inequality of evolutionary achievement, privilege and abilities. The fact of a hierarchical Universe forces us to be aware of our own process of judging value. A fully healthy person will have a value system which is in harmony with the hierarchy of the Universe. Such a person will be totally in touch with their inner purpose (spirit), and they radiate health on the physical, emotional, mental and moral level. This, as we have seen, is described in Stanza 9,and is a definition of health.

One of the most important parts of training to be a homœopathic healer is to develop insight and understanding of yourself and others and the natural processes of life and health.

The physical body can be divided into two:

VITAL BODY
CHEMICAL BODY

Diagram 2

The chemical body is the vehicle that we inhabit, it is animated by the vitality which enters at conception and leaves at the death of the physical body.

> *The material organism, without the Vital Force, is capable of no sensation, no function, no self-preservation; it derives all sensation and performs all the functions of life solely by means of the immaterial being (the Vital Force) which animates the material organism in health and in disease.*
>
> *(Stanza 10)*

It is well known that strong emotions can change at once the normal state of our physical body. A sudden fright or shock produces a 'flight or fight' response in the body involving drastic physical changes. However, this kind of process goes on not only in the face of emergencies but all the time. In fact, the state of our physical body, its shape, the way it functions, its state of health and disease, is being moulded all the time by our emotional and our mental state. For example, persistent feelings or emotions like jealousy, anger and humiliation will eventually produce changes in our physical body which accurately reflect these negative emotions. Such changes are called physical or gross pathology. Persistent negative thought patterns or misconceptions about the world will also change our bodies. These processes are in conformity with natural law regarding the hierarchy of power in the life process.

There are two links which bring about this process of change in the physical body:
1. The secretions of the ductless glands
2. The nervous system

These two form a link between the mind and the emotions on one part and the physical body on the other part by communicating messages to all areas of the body.

THE DUCTLESS GLANDS

There are six main ductless glands; the pineal which is located in the cranial cavity, the pituitary, also in the skull behind the third eye position, the thyroid in the throat, the thymus in the chest, the adrenals, one above each kidney and the gonads (ovaries and testes). Each of these glands is associated with a Chakra or centre of energy. The qualities of these Chakras sum up the influences which affect the secretions from the associated ductless gland. Diagram 3 (overleaf) shows the main glands, centres and their main associations. Much knowledge of the causes of disease and the pathways to health is contained in the study of these centres.

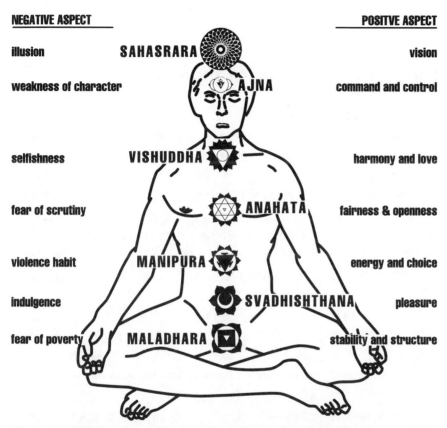

NEGATIVE ASPECT		POSITVE ASPECT
illusion	SAHASRARA	vision
weakness of character	AJNA	command and control
selfishness	VISHUDDHA	harmony and love
fear of scrutiny	ANAHATA	fairness & openness
violence habit	MANIPURA	energy and choice
indulgence	SVADHISHTHANA	pleasure
fear of poverty	MALADHARA	stability and structure

**The seven principle centres which focus the qualities and characteristics of our nature.
We progress by developing the positive side of each centre or Chakra.**

Diagram 3

The breath is a further link between mind, emotions and body; the rate and manner of breathing reflects mental and emotional states. A regulated, balanced breath will ensure a calm mental and emotional presence.

We can now begin to see the forces which determine the state of health and of disease. Health is order in the human economy, disease is disorder or disharmony. Positive thoughts and emotions establish order and health in the human economy.

1.3 TO CURE OR NOT TO CURE

The question is often asked whether it is wrong to seek to remove suffering since suffering is a sign of change and development. We are on earth, it is argued, to struggle to improve ourselves.

It is true that we have purposes and if we do not pursue our purposes we become ill and unhappy. We need to recognise that conflicts and difficulties are often necessary to keep us in touch with our purpose. Those regimes, methods and health programmes which offer formulae for health and happiness that claim to remove illnesses or avoid the need to suffer problems and conflicts are doubly bad; first being false, and second they give additional problems of negative feelings when they do not work. What tends to happen is either we fail to keep to the prescribed rules and feel guilty, or we keep to them and when we fail we will either blame ourselves for being inadequate or those that made the promises. In fact, any existing negative thought will be reinforced. Constructive medicine helps us see the next step we need to take and frees us to achieve this. Disease and health are states existing along the same spectrum of being; our state of being reflects how successful we are at living our lives. To complain about our diseases is to boast of our own shortcomings.

We may do one of three things in response to a pain. Firstly we can ignore it and hope it will go away, and initially it may do so. Secondly we can suppress or hide the pain by hindering the body's natural response to the cause of the pain, for example by taking painkillers. Third we can seek the cause of the pain and deal with that so that the pain is removed in its entirety. We no longer need it. These three alternatives apply to any disease from sea-sickness to cancer and AIDS.

1.4 THE VITAL FORCE

Hahnemann uses the word 'Lebenskraft' meaning strength to live and also the term 'dynamis' or 'spirit-like Vital Force'. This is clearly expressed in Stanza 9, (page 4).

Health is not only the perfect functioning of all the parts plus a sense of general well-being, it also involves a sense of belonging and a sense of purpose. The ability of individuals to fulfil their potential and develop their qualities through life so as to be more evolved at death is a necessary part of health. This will also enhance the good of the whole, since each one of us becomes a positive part of the Universe in our own unique way. The worst thing we can try to do is to 'change' someone, to 'improve' them or to fit them into any 'mould' like a belief, creed or cult – we must leave people free to develop along their own individual path, meeting their own needs and developing their own unique qualities.

1.5 DISEASE

Disease reflects a failure to develop the individual potential or purpose of life. Disease manifests on any level when the Vital Force is unable to fully maintain perfect health. The Vital Force is the innate intelligence which strives to restore health, it is the 'dynamis' referred to in The Organon. The immune system is just one tool used by the Vital Force to constantly restore us to optimum health. The move towards health is a constant throwing outwards of disease, moving it away from the more vital functions and parts. The disease process strives constantly to move inwards towards important levels and more vital organs. As our best defence procedures become impaired so we become more diseased.

There is another part of us called the Conscious Force. This is our choosing self. We choose to do things from habit, which includes individual, cultural or social habits which may not be good for our whole life's purposes and needs. Our habits, mental, emotional and physical, may persistently undermine our ability to be healthy and to evolve. We may choose to act against the requirements of good health on any of the four levels; physical, emotional, mental or spiritual. The Vital Force will strive constantly to minimise and repair the ill-effects of harmful choices and constantly gives us the best health we can attain – given our state of health.

This model of health and disease gives us our fourth principle.

PRINCIPLE IV

The responsibility for our health rests on the choices we make or fail to make and what we seek from medical help is advice and guidance as to what these choices are and how to make them. Medical treatment should help us in this process and not seek to help us avoid these choices.

1.6 THE DIRECTION OF CURE

It follows from this model of health and disease that we cause our diseases ourselves by our own choices in life. If we have cancer our own Vital Force has created it for us and it is the best possible thing we can have given our state of health as a whole. The Vital Force acts according to natural laws. If we understand these laws and conform to them, ie work with them, we will achieve health and happiness. This gives us a tremendous potential for cure by looking at ourselves to understand why we have our present illness and how we need to change to cure it. Healers, counsellors, therapists and homœopaths can all play their part in helping us in this process towards health

---

PRINCIPLE V

There is a natural direction of cure, which is that healing takes place from within outwards, from above downwards, from a vital organ to a less important organ, and in the reverse order of appearance.

---

1. From within outwards. During the healing process, disease will move outwards and away from the heart centre. This includes a movement down the limbs and out from the fingers and toes, and into the neck and head and out at the scalp.
2. From the more vital and important organs to the less; and from the higher levels to the lower levels. This includes mental and emotional symptoms changing for physical symptoms and organ dysfunction. Also from the inner, more vital, organs to the outer, eg from the kidneys to the bladder.
3. Sensation should normally become less severe and more readily tolerated as the disease process is reversed. There may be a temporary increase in the disease sensation or pain which quickly gives way to an amelioration. This is known as homœopathic aggravation which is discussed in detail later.
4. Past symptoms may recur in their reverse order. If any previous illnesses did not abate from a correct curative process of dealing with their true cause they will recur as a part of the healing process. They will however recur in their 'reverse order of coming', so the latest illness will be cured first and the first to have been suffered will manifest itself again last. These recurrences of old diseases, in their reverse order, are a sign of a true healing process. Not all past ailments need recur only those that have not been correctly and fully cured by the Vital Force.

It is so that lesser diseases abate in the presence of newer more acute or more serious diseases. When the newer more serious disease is cured, the older disease will reappear. It is unlikely that diseases which have been treated by conventional drugs or operations even though they have abated are in fact correctly cured. It is most likely that they have been suppressed. These so called 'cured' diseases will recur in the organism once a correct healing process has begun. They will manifest again in their reverse order of coming. These returning illnesses are almost always less in intensity, severity and duration, but occasionally they may be life-threatening and the physician must be prepared to give careful and correct treatment of these disease states. For example, if a patient had a pneumonia in the past which was treated with conventional drugs, the prescriber should be prepared for this to recur as part of a true healing process, and may also warn the patient of this possibility. Correct and prompt homœopathic treatment will be required in such cases.

1.7 THE REQUIREMENTS FOR HEALTH

PHYSICAL HEALTH The first requirement is fresh and nutritious food and clean water. The continued use of refined and processed food is unhealthy, and likewise the over-use of stimulants and drugs, including coffee, alcohol, cigarettes, etc, is detrimental to the health. Food which involves disrespect of the source, whether it is the cruelty involved in rearing battery hens, or by the use of artificial fertilizers or from over-fishing, etc, produces unhealthy food. We must kill to live, it is in the order of things. However, how our vegetables and animals live is most important, as is how they die. The issue of vegetarianism is an individual choice. It is the author's belief that meat eaters can be healthy if they show a conscience for the quality of the life and death of the creatures they eat.

A reasonable amount of recreation and relaxation is necessary to health, as is sufficient sleep. Exercise is necessary to maintain a healthy body, and a healthy attitude to sex is important for our well-being. Quantities cannot be put on any of these things, since our first principle for health is that all individuals are different and so their need for each of these requirements differ. It is possible to over-indulge in food or drink, take soft drugs, do without sleep, avoid or over use sex, eat junk food, all of these – for a time; but for a time only. How long you can get away with it differs for each individual. All of these things are however detrimental in the long term. Failings on the physical level like smoking or eating refined food can be compensated for by a strong, healthy and happy emotional and mental attitude to these matters. Equally, virtues on the bodily level can be totally undermined by negative emotions and mental attitudes. Any guilt associated with healthy appetites in sex or daily living will be a powerful drain on health which can be much worse than a failing on the physical level. The human mind is the most powerful thing yet evolved and created by the Universe.

EMOTIONAL HEALTH Sexual needs are an expression of our emotional state and we need to have a degree of satisfaction in the sexual sphere, although this will vary from person to person. For emotional health we need support and companionship from friends, family and partners. We need to be able to express our feelings, to develop our emotional awareness and to recognize the range of emotions and recognise when positive emotions become negative. Trust, support, love and expression are needed for emotional health.

The modern scientific model of the world has been based solely on its material manifestation. The adoption of this model in conventional medicine has proved to be disastrous. Our emotional needs are equally as important as our needs on the physical and other levels. What makes us unique is a combination of different personality traits, our cultural backgrounds, our physical make-up, our talents and life experiences. However, what makes us ill is the same for all of us; we all need to be loved and to love, and we all need to have something that gives our life meaning. Without these we lose health.

In the western world today, most of our illness stems from a failure to give emotional guidance and encourage healthy emotional expression at puberty. Society decrees that mental exercise and work predominate throughout adolescence, when the emotions are burgeoning and needing education and direction. As a result, emotional causes of disease predominate in our society.

If we do not know how to give and receive love freely, we keep these needs secret. Because the body and psyche requires these emotional needs to be met, it will force us to have 'hidden agendas' to try to manipulate circumstances and people so that some of our needs are received. This activity leads to all sorts of fustrations, disappointments, misunderstandings and hurt; and all these in turn lead to more emotional disease.

MENTAL HEALTH The requirements of mental health are:
1. A pattern of positive thoughts.
2. To discipline the mind by developing its qualities. These include memory, logic, analysis and imagination.
3. To clear the mind of negative anxieties and worries; first by learning to recognize them, then by changing them to their positive opposites.

If we feed our minds on a diet of negativity it will becomes diseased. It is useful to censor unnecessary negative influences so that we view, read and hear uplifting and inspiring things. The brain needs to be encouraged not to dwell on negative thoughts. There are many books and practices to help us achieve a calm, clear, retentive and positive mind. (Some references are given at the end of this Chapter).

SPIRITUAL (MORAL) HEALTH As medical practitioners we need to be able to judge what is health and what is disease on all four levels we have mentioned. Health on this highest level is:
1. Having a clear insight into right and wrong.
2. Having a sense of belonging.
3. Having a sense of purpose.

This involves having a sense of good which goes beyond the natural animal instinct of survival, ie good for me, for my family, my group, my tribe, my nation, my race; it is a greater awareness of good for the four kingdoms – mineral, vegetable, animal and human – and, in fact, good for the whole Universe. This is what is meant by service, and a sense of this is required for moral and spiritual health. A disease which often stems from dissatisfaction on the spiritual level in modern times is depression, this is because it has become difficult to have a sense of belonging in an increasingly fragmented society. Without a sense of belonging it is also difficult to have a sense of purpose.

1.8 THE HIERARCHY OF SACRIFICE

The organism may sacrifice an organ to ensure the survival of the whole. This would be an expression of the best 'Defence Posture'.

The normal channels of elimination work to keep the organism healthy. On a physical level they are, the bowels, the kidneys and the lungs – corresponding to the elements of earth, water and air respectively. The menstrual flow and perspiration correspond to fire. All these discharges provide an external route for the process of cleansing. Elimination must also occur on the emotional and mental level to remain in health. This is why it is so important to stay in touch with and express our emotions, positive and negative, so that they do not build up and stagnate.

Toxic overload can result from not observing the requirements for health on all levels.

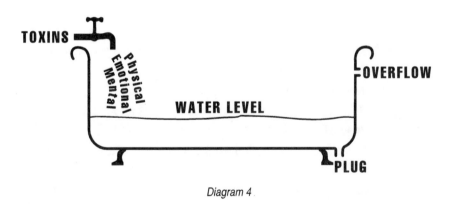

Diagram 4

In this diagram the plug represents the five physical channels of cleansing mentioned above. There are many things that may reduce their efficiency, for example, the use of anti-perspirants, being constipated, taking the birth-control pill, etc

The overflow will be used when the body needs to throw out toxins with an extra effort. This process includes colds, catarrh, coughs and any minor acute illnesses which continue for a while, do their job, and then end.

When the toxin level is too high for the plug hole and the overflow to cope with the bath reaches its total capacity and overflows into chronic illness. Catarrhal difficulties, sinusitis or rhinitis all the year round, eczema, rheumatism, gout, anxieties, neurosis, depression and all chronic illness can now be perceived. The location, type and depth of the illness will depend on each individual's state of being (of health). Health is more dependent on the internal state than on any external influences. Each one of us will have a weak link either hereditary, a past accident, a past illness not resolved properly or anything which blocks our healing energy, on any level. A love disappointment, a bereavement, a humiliation or unhappy or traumatic childhood experiences; these can all mark a pattern of ill health and disease upon us, until we learn how to balance and heal them.

1.9 HOW DISEASE ARISES

Every trauma will affect us on all levels:
1. The ductless glands react, their secretions are altered and repercussions on the emotional level follow.
2. The mind reacts and our thoughts are changed.
3. The physical body is affected; organs and systems and the processes of cleansing may all be affected.

There is an interaction between all the parts of the body, the mind and the emotions.

There is also an interaction between the person and the environment. Groups of cells form an organ on the next level up, eg the kidney. Groups of organs form yet another group, eg the urinary system. The groups of bodily systems form the whole person who in turn belongs to other groups, like families, races, planets or solar systems. Within the smaller groupings we find yet more smaller groups like atoms, molecules, neutrons, etc. Activity by certain groups which causes discomfort or harm to other groups creates unharmonious conditions which upset the delicate balance of self-preservation activity. Health is when a being is in harmony with the various parts of their environment. Disease is when disharmony disrupts activity designed to restore harmony. Healing is activity designed to remove the disharmony and to restore the natural order of peace and health.

Evolution is a natural process of change to further the greater purpose – the purpose of the group on the next level up. Adaptability to these changes is a sign of health. The survival of the physical body is not always essential or possible to the restoration of health in the context of 'the best possible health posture on all levels' a fact which becomes clearer as old age approaches. In his book "The Science of Homœopathy", George Vithoulkas says:

"On the other hand if there is a disturbance on the mental/spiritual plane, the person's very existence is threatened. This is seen in conditions such as senility, schizophrenia and imbecility. Although the physical body is the medium through which higher faculties can manifest themselves in this material world, it's maintainance cannot become an end in itself. It is doubtful that anyone would claim that people have come into this life just to eat, to enjoy sex and to acquire money and possessions. Even the most primitive men see a higher goal in life, leading them to value faith (which is a degree of understanding) and love; take these things away from even the most primitive person and the will to live will be lost."

When we have an infection it is because the internal conditions have changed, the local environment is now attractive to bacteria or other organisms which come and set up processes that are fitting to the new environment. This process is actually beneficial to the process of healing. It is harmful to kill such organisms of infection with chemical agents like antibiotics, antifungals etc, without changing the environment; when you change the conditions the organisms will go.

1.10 THE MEANING OF SYMPTOMS

If disease is an activity designed to restore health then disease symptoms must be beneficial. Symptoms come from within. External events and trauma may initiate a process leading to illness, but each individual's reaction to the trauma is vitally important and is unique. Take the simplest case of an accidental cut with a knife. The knife is at once removed and plays no part in what follows: there is redness (Latin RUBOR), pain (DOLOR), swelling (TUMOR) and heat (COLOR). All these local symptoms are produced by the body's defence system. There is also an emotional reaction ranging from indifference to hysteria (both unhealthy) and all the reactions that can lie between. Also, there will be a mental reaction, for example, thoughts of how to avoid such accidents, blame and regret, etc. Thus nothing happens on one level without there being repercussions on all other levels.

Similarly a love disappointment can produce symptoms on the physical level, such as headaches, tiredness, nausea, etc, as well as emotional and mental symptoms. Moral peccadillos likewise can produce emotional and mental symptoms. Much religious teaching emphasises this. My favourite example is the YAMAS and NIYAMAS of Yoga, which teach that moral rectitude will produce the necessary foundation for a healthy mind, body and soul. (See notes to this chapter)

THE UNITY OF THE PARTS

Our various models and diagrams of mankind serve to help us to a greater understanding but they should not lead us away from the fact of unity. Our being is a single whole entity, all of which is affected by any change or influence on any part. (Principle I)

1.11 SUSCEPTIBILITY

Why do some people go down with a disease when others do not? Why this particular disease? Why are there epidemics? Why does vaccination seriously harm some children and not others? Susceptibility is the ability of a person to have disease and determines which particular disease they have. It is a well known observation that immunity and vulnerability varies between individuals, families, races and other groups. The modern world has externalised everything, from God to the cause of the common cold/infection. Our 'soil' is what allows illness to grow and also determines it's particular individual nature. What is our state of being? How healthy are we? Where on the spectrum of health and disease are we located? What causes have brought us to the state of health and disease we now enjoy and how have we earned this state? These questions can be answered by a study of this concept of susceptibility. (See Chapter 2)

1.12 CAUSES OF DISEASE

Our Vital Force and its ability to keep us healthy and creative depends on how much it has to contend with. The first cause of potential ill health is what is inherited. Our inheritance forms a major part of our state of health. It is observed that certain illness have strong inheritable weaknesses, tuberculosis and venereal disease are examples. If in both parents there is a serious organ weakness, eg kidney disease, the child will frequently inherit this weakness.

There are causes which are 'thrust upon us'; we may be born into a war time environment, or we may suffer earthquakes, etc. It may be postulated that our greater needs have brought us into all of these situations, but for practical purposes they are thrust upon us by external, larger events.

Our Conscious Choosing Force can now bring upon us acquired causes of illness. We can acquire weaknesses by exposing ourselves to bad habits on the emotional and mental planes as well as the physical.

A special note is needed to cover the case where children who are 'in trust' to their parents and guardians find themselves under the care of the corrupt and misguided. This and other similar situations gives the opportunity for people to create illness and unhappiness.

Disease, then, is a subtle form of disharmony and disorder where the purpose of life is not being fully pursued.

PRINCIPLE VI
Symptoms of disease are desirable manifestations of the body's own intelligent efforts to maintain health.

1.13 MEDICINE

A medicine is an agent applied to remove the symptoms of disease. If you believe that disease comes from outside, then you will strive to destroy these outside agencies. Similarly, if you believe that symptoms are undesirable manifestations of hostile outside influences, you will seek to remove and destroy them. Both of these beliefs and courses of action are contrary to the view of the world, mankind and the nature of health and disease given above. Contrary to the orthodox view we have:

PRINCIPLE VII
Health is more dependent on the internal state of our susceptibility than on any external influences.

1.14 THE DYNAMIC NATURE OF DISEASE

We have seen that disease can be caused on any level of the human system.

We have seen that disease on one level can and does produce symptoms on all the other levels of our being.

Therefore, this disease process must be subtle enough to permeate our thoughts, feelings, energy pattern, nerves, glands, organs and cells and to the very foundations of our being. The nature of such a process we call 'DYNAMIC'. We see then that disease is caused and therefore must be cured in this kind of dynamic way.

> *When a person falls ill, it is only this spiritual, self acting (automatic) Vital Force, everywhere present in his organism, that is primarily deranged by the dynamic influence upon it of a morbific agent inimical to life; it is only the vital principle, deranged to such an abnormal state, that can furnish the organism with its disagreeable sensations, and incline it to the irregular processes which we call disease; ...which...only makes itself known by morbid symptoms, and in no other way can it make itself known.*
>
> *(Stanza 11)*

> *Our Vital Force, as a spirit-like dynamis, cannot be attacked and affected by injurious influences... otherwise than in a spirit-like (dynamic) way, and in like manner, all such morbid derangements (diseases) cannot be removed from it by the physician in any other way than by the spirit-like (dynamic virtual) alternative powers of the serviceable medicines.*
>
> *(Stanza 16)*

Chapter 1 notes

THE FOUR KINGDOMS

I would like you to consider why human beings benefit from medicines drawn from the four kingdoms of nature. Remember our original premise that we all belong to the same Universe, each individual part or group having a purpose in this meaningful whole.

Look at the qualities of the four kingdoms and learn to relate these to individual needs:

1. THE MINERAL has only structure and no observable vitality. It is passive and inert and moves only by external forces. Minerals develop structure with order. The highest, most structured mineral form is the crystal, (and once a stable form is developed vitality will be engendered). This stage relates to the skeleton of man.

2. THE VEGETABLE has structure and vitality. It can move and respond to changes in the physical environment. It can organise matter to its own purpose. This corresponds to the fleshly body in which man is active, dynamic and vital. Energy is needed to sustain the form.

3. THE ANIMAL has structure, vitality, and develops emotional response to its environment. It has a passive mind and limited memory. Only the species as a whole has individuality; within the species all are alike. The group spirit (species) rules, responds and adapts.

4. THE HUMAN has structure, vitality, develops emotional responsiveness and is developing the individual active mind. The human mind is the most powerful thing yet evolved. It is capable of both concrete thought and abstract thought. More advanced humans are able to open up even higher qualities of the mind (creative thought) and all of us are capable of spiritual awareness.

HIERARCHIES OF IMPORTANCE

Suggested hierarchies of importance from highest to lowest:

I VEHICLES

1. Spiritual level
2. Mental level
3. Emotional level
4. Physical level

II BODILY SYSTEMS

1. The brain and the central nervous system
2. The glandular system
   a) ductless glands
   b) lymphatic system
3. The heart and circulation
4. The lungs and respiration
5. The digestive system and main abdominal organs
6. The elimination system
   a) kidneys and bladder
   b) large intestine and bowel
   c) sweat glands and perspiration
7. The reproductive system
8. The locomotor and peripheral nervous system
9. The sensory organs

III ORGANS

1. The brain
2. The heart
3. The liver

4. The lungs
5. The kidneys
6. The spleen
7. The pancreas

THE EIGHT LIMBS OF YOGA

Patanjali, an ancient Indian sage, co-ordinated the systems of Yoga and wrote his famous Sutras (or notes) putting forward the philosophy and practices of Yoga more than 2,000 years ago. In the second chapter are to be found the eight 'limbs' of Yoga, the first two of which are:

YAMAS   ie Conduct towards others
                AHIMSA – non violence
                SATYA – truthfulness
                ASTEYA – abstention from theft
                BRAHMACHARYA – abstention from sexual misconduct
                APARIGRAHA – abstention from greed

NIYAMAS   ie Observances
                SAUCHA – purity
                SANTOSHA – contentment
                TAPAS – abstention from materialism
                SVADHYAYA – study
                ISVARA PRANIDHANA – devotion to God

Observation of these precepts of daily living give a firm foundation upon which to build spiritual endeavour and higher development. They offer peace and freedom from troubles in the world.

EXERCISES

1. What is health? What is disease?
2. What is a symptom and why are they produced?
3. What do you understand by the word "cure"?
4. What do you need to know when a patient tells you they have a pain?

RECOMMENDED READING FOR CHAPTER 1

Bach, Edward 'Heal Thyself'

Close, Stuart 'The Genius of Homœopathy', Chapters 5, 6, 9

Diamond 'Fit for Life.' and 'Living Health'

Gutman, W. 'Homœopathy', Chapters 1-5

Harrison, John 'Love your Disease

Hahnemann, Samuel, 'The Organon of Medicine', Stanzas 1-82, 201-203

Hay, Louise 'You Can Heal Your Life'

Kent, James Tyler, 'Lectures on Homœopathic Philosophy' Chapters 1, 2, 4, 8, 9, 12, 14

Myss, Caroline and Shealy, CN 'The Creation of Health'

Ohsawa, George 'Zen Macrobiotics' and 'The Book of Judgement'

Rendle, Peter 'The Chakras'

Roberts, Herbert 'The Principles, Art and Science of Homeopathy' Chapters 1-7

Vithoulkas, George 'The Science of Homœopathy' Chapters 1-10

Vithoulkas, George 'Medicine of the New Man'

Wright Hubbard, Elizabeth, 'A Brief Study Course in Homœopathy' Chapters 1, 2, 14

Chapter II

A PROFILE OF DISEASE

1. Categories of Disease
2. Symptoms – What are they?
3. Causes
4. What is to be cured
5. Provings
6. Potentisation – Dynamic Medicines
7. Similars – an empirical law
8. Enhancing symptoms
9. Suppression
10. Principles VIII IX and X
11. Exercises
12. Recommended Reading

2.1 CATEGORIES OF DISEASE

We can distinguish three categories of disease; first-aid, acute and chronic:

FIRST-AID means the application of remedies both internally and externally to illness, pain or discomfort, arising from external forces or trauma at the time these happen. The most common first-aid needs arise from knocks, falls, insect stings, burns and scalds. Food poisoning and travel sickness/diarrhoea come under this category although individual susceptibility will govern their incidence:

> *Those so-called local maladies which have been pro-*
> *duced a short time previously, solely by an external*
> *lesion, still appear at first sight to deserve the name of*
> *local diseases. But then the lesion must be very trivial,*
> *and in that case it would be of no great moment. For*
> *in the case of injuries accruing to the body from with-*
> *out, if they be at all severe, the whole living organism*
> *sympathizes; there occur fever, etc. The treatment of*
> *such diseases is relegated to surgery; but this is right*
> *only in so far as the affected parts require mechanical*
> *aid, whereby the external obstacles to the cure, (which*
> *can only be expected to take place by the agency of*
> *the Vital Force), may be removed by mechanical*
> *means, eg by the reduction of dislocations...*
>
> *(Stanza 186)*

We also include in first-aid emotional trauma like fright, shock or grief at their time of impact. However, after a few hours or a day or so any remaining effects of emotional trauma must be viewed as an acute illness or even as a chronic disease symptom. This time limit is equally true of any first-aid trauma like a fall, cut or travel diarrhoea. If any symptoms remain we say the patient has never been well since the incident. The reason why symptoms or diseases remain after an accident of one kind or another is because of weakness in the constitution, or to put it another way, because of the susceptibility of the patient.

ACUTE ILLNESS is one that has an inherent tendency to end. The disease comes on, rises to a peak then declines. It is true that some serious acute illness can end in death, but either way the illness comes to an end within a certain time.

There can be sequelae, or after-conditions, following some acute illnesses, some of these are well known, eg impotency after mumps. These after-effects vary from person to person according to their susceptibility or strength of constitution and this comes under the heading of chronic disease. Acute illness may be slow or rapid in its onset and progress but it will clear up without any consequences remaining.

Many individuals suffer a chronic state of illness which has from time to time an acute flare up, this is called sub-acute illness. For example, a person may get seasonal hay fever, or asthma attacks only on violent exertion or in certain weather conditions. These are sometimes termed periodic lesions. The term lesions originally meant an injury but is now applied to all disease changes in organs or tissues, (gross pathology as opposed to subtle pathology in mental or emotional functions).

CHRONIC ILLNESS The Vital Force in this situation is unable to either cure the disease or let go of the physical body in death. There is an ongoing and unresolved battle with disease moving ever inward towards the more vital parts and levels while the healing force is striving to minimise the disease by constantly 'externalising' it. Let us recall now that changes on any one level will have repercussions on all other levels, where adjustments have to be made.

There are also two further categories of disease to consider:

ENDEMIC DISEASE is found in certain localities or in certain races. Malaria is endemic to areas of stagnant water. Cholera may spread wide in an epidemic but it is endemic to certain parts of Asia. Certain blood cell diseases are widely found only in certain racial groups, eg sickle cell anaemia in Afro-Caribbean peoples.

EPIDEMIC DISEASE is a widespread outbreak amongst a large number of people in any locality.

Susceptibility to disease depends on many factors which we discuss in section 8 of this chapter. There are some things to which we are all susceptible to, eg a bullet in the brain. Many of us can become susceptible by frequent exposure to certain adverse conditions, this gives rise to endemic suscepti- bility. We can find large groups of people susceptible to the same disease at any one time – epidemic susceptibility. The interesting question to ask about such a virulent acute epidemic disease as the Black Death is why one third of the population did not die of it?

2.2 WHAT ARE SYMPTOMS?

Symptoms are the expression of disease in the human economy. A symptom is a change in normal comfortable functioning of bodily systems and organs; or a change in normal qualities of mind like memory, understanding and will; or a change in normal emotional expression and reaction. Symptoms vary in intensity and frequency. Where do symptoms first show?

> It is the morbidly affected vital energy alone that produces dis-
> ease so that the morbid phenomena perceptible to our senses
> express at the same time all the internal change, that is to say,
> the whole morbid derangement of the internal dynamis;
>
> (Stanza 12)

This is saying that disease begins with inner disturbance of the inner energy level of the vitality; it has a dynamic cause (see I.14). Hahnemann goes on to say here that all this inner change in health is clearly shown by symptoms "perceptible to our senses" which "reveal the whole disease".

To use another model we can describe our whole human being as having a state of health/disease. This is a state of being which reflects our progress through life using all we have been given by inheritance, external forces, and also what has been acquired. Let us call this our Central State of Health (CS).

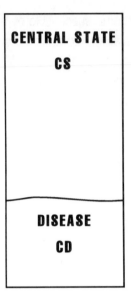

CENTRAL STATE

CS

The disease is the disturbance in
the Central State called Central
Disturbance, CD.

DISEASE

CD

Diagram 5

When we become ill, the occasion, timing and nature of the illness will all
have reasons and causes discernible to the trained observer. Illness may
occur, but the Vital Force will limit its expression to trivial minor symptoms for
as long as it can. For example, there may for some time exist a degree of
absent mindedness, a degree of irresolution, some weepiness at slight
causes, a few spots, occasional colds or a chronic mild catarrh.

These illnesses may be referred to as Peripheral Disturbances. Note that
they are outward manifestations of an internal state of less than perfect
health.

> *The affection of the morbidly deranged, spirit-like dynamis*
> *(Vital Force) that animates our body in the invisible interior,*
> *and the totality of the outwardlycognizable symptoms produced*
> *by it in the organism and representing the existing malady,*
> *constitute a whole; they are one and the same.*
>
> *(Stanza 15)*

And yet very little reflection will suffice to convince us that no external malady (not occasioned by some important injury from without) can arise, persist or even grow worse without some internal cause, without the co-operation of the whole organism, which consequently must be in a diseased state. It could not make its appearance at all without the consent of the whole of the rest of the health, and without the participation of the rest of the living whole (of the Vital Force that pervades all the other sensitive and irritable parts of the organism): indeed, it is impossible to conceive its production without the instrumentality of the whole (deranged) life; so intimately are all parts of the organism connected together to form an individual whole in sensations and functions. No eruption on the lips, no whitlow can occur without previous and simultaneous internal ill-health.

(Stanza 189)

We therefore always have two parts to disease: the Central Disturbance to Health and the Peripheral Disturbance (PD), portrayed thus:

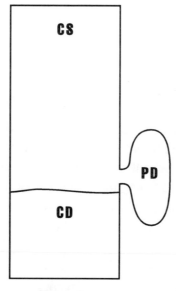

Diagram 6

Disease is the sum of the Central Disturbance and the Peripheral Disturbance.

When does the Vital Force find it necessary to put the Central Disturbance into a symptom or group of symptoms called disease? To return to our bath tub model we can see that eventually the toxic load from mental, emotional, or physical sources, will rise beyond the level which the Vital Force can contain and Peripheral Disease (lesions) will manifest; the bath tub overflows its capacity. This threshold level, at which lesions become evident varies with each individual and will depend upon their history and state of health.

> It is evident that man's Vital Force, when encumbered with a chronic disease which it is unable to overcome instinctively by its own powers, adopts the plan of developing a local malady on some external part, solely for this object, that by making and keeping in a diseased state this part which is not indispensable to human life, it may thereby silence the internal disease, which otherwise threatens to destroy the vital organs (and to deprive the patient of life.
>
> *(Stanza 201)*

2.3 CAUSES

There is always an Exciting Cause which you will find, on close examination tipped the balance past the threshold level. It may be an acute illness, ill-conceived medical treatment, a vaccination, an accident, a love disappointment, a bereavement or a fright. Here again we observe 'a never been well since' situation. The underlying internal cause which is reflected in the Central Disturbance is the true Fundamental Cause of chronic disease. This is the susceptible state of health.

MAINTAINING CAUSES There can frequently exist a cause of ill health which for the time being cannot be removed, for example unhealthy or unsatisfactory living or working conditions, a sick relative to be nursed, and emotional causes which the body suffers from, diseases which:

*Originated and are kept up by emotional causes, such as con-
tinued anxiety, worry, vexation, wrongs and the frequent occurrence of great fear and fright. This kind of emotional diseases
in time destroys the corporal health, often to a great degree.*

(Stanza 225)

You may have to visit a patient's home or workplace or meet their spouse
before you become aware of a maintaining cause.

Refer to Chapter 1 where three causes of disease were given as inherited, those thrust upon us and those acquired. These causes all contribute to
the fundamental cause, which is the soil of our individual susceptibility to
'catch' disease. (This subject will be discussed in more detail in Chapter 4 on
miasms.)

2.4 WHAT IS TO BE CURED

It is necessary to know what is to be cured. Is it the Peripheral Disease or
diseases? Is it the Central Disturbance? How can we distinguish these? It is
not only necessary to know what to cure, it is also necessary to know how to
apply the correct curative method. It is necessary to know how to identify and
remove any obstacles to cure on the superficial and deeper levels.

*If the physician clearly perceives what is to be cured in diseases,
that is to say, in every individual case of disease …if he clearly
perceives what is curative in medicines, that is to say, in each
individual medicine… and if he knows how to adapt, according
to clearly defined principles, what is curative in medicines to
what he has discovered to be undoubtedly morbid in the
patient, so that the recovery must ensue …and if, finally, he
knows the obstacles to recovery in each case and is aware how
to remove them so that the restoration may be permanent, then
he understands how to treat judiciously and rationally, and he
is a true practitioner of the healing art.*

(Stanza 3)

Symptoms tell us about the nature of the illness. Refer to Stanza 11 where it states, "by morbid symptoms alone and in no other way does disease make itself known to us."

Symptoms therefore are the (desirable) outward expression of an illness. Their cause lies in a disturbance of the Central State where they originated and express the person's best possible defence posture. Should we seek to remove a symptom or group of symptoms disregarding the reason for their being there and without attending to their true inner cause we put the person into a second best (inferior) defence posture. This mode of treatment is termed 'suppression'.

> But those affections, alterations and ailments appearing on the external parts that do not arise from any external injury or that have only some slight external wound for their immediate exciting cause, are produced in quite another manner; their source lies in some internal malady. To consider them as mere local affections, and at the same time to treat them only, or almost only, as it were surgically, with topical application or other similar remedies – as the old school has done from the remotest ages – is as absurd as it is pernicious in its results.
>
> (Stanza 187)

2.5 PROVINGS

The foundation of the homœopathic system lies in the method of proving remedies or medicinal agents. To produce a proving small groups of normally healthy people are given the same substance repeatedly until symptoms appear. Dangerous or lethal symptoms are obtained from records of poisonings. The proving is stopped by antidote when symptoms become too troublesome to bear. The symptoms from various provers are carefully arranged in significant order to make up a coherent picture covering the physical, emotional and mental levels. In this way we have today many hundreds of properly proven drug pictures. Stanza 3 quoted above says "...the physician... clearly perceives what is curative in medicines..." and this is achieved by these careful provings which make our medicines scientific in that we know from experience exactly what our medicines can both cause and cure.

PRINCIPLE VIII
Properly conducted provings of single medicinal drugs given to healthy human beings provides homœopathy with knowledge of the action of the medicines in our Materia Medica.

2.6 POTENTISATION

The use of crude medicinal drugs soon gave way in Hahnemann's work to 'potentised' medicines. Potentisation is a method of releasing the deeper energy of the essential medicine. The process has three parts.

Firstly dilution in a relatively inert substance, either a mixture of alcohol and pure water or sac lac (sugar extracted from milk).

Secondly trituration (grinding) and thirdly succussion (banging) of the substance. In the case of metals, other minerals and hard seeds or nuts, the substance is ground down in a succession of stages each involving dilution with an inert substance. In the case of plant juices and other easily dissolved medicines these are diluted in liquid and succussed. As an example, one measure of the medicine is placed in 99 measures of the inert substance, this is then succussed many times. The second step is to put one measure of this mixture into 99 measures of inert substance and repeat the succussion. This process is repeated again, each repetition raising the potency once. If this is repeated 30 times we have a 30c potency. After 12c, according to Avogadro's Law, there is none of the original substance left in the diluted medicine, but the potent energy with the pattern of the full drug picture contained within it exists in the potentised liquid which is now termed Dynamic. The implications of this process are several:

1. We now have a dynamic medicine which is capable of treating the dynamic nature of disease (see Chapter 1.14).
2. We can use poisons or disease products like the discharge of tuberculosis, for example, or any kind of noxious or dangerous substances which are all rendered both harmless and immensely potent medicines by this paradox of potentisation, a paradox which is alchemical in nature.
3. We can, by raising potencies, treat disease which is deep both in the patient (even inherited factors can be changed) and in the disease pathology.

So that now we have in Homœopathy:

> "...specific, therapeutic instruments for effecting their certain and permanent cure." and "From such a Materia Medica everything that is conjectural, all that is mere assertion or imaginary should be strictly excluded; everything should be the pure language of nature carefully and honestly interrogated."
> (Stanza 143 and 144)

Homœopathic remedies are made from substances in all the four kingdoms, mineral, vegetable (medicinal herbs), animal eg. snake venom and human. Remedies taken from the human kingdom are disease products called Nosodes, for example, Tuberculinum is a remedy made from the discharge of patients with active TB.

Homœopaths today mostly use decimal(x),centesimal(c), millesimal(M) and fifty millesimal(LM) potencies.

2.7 SIMILARS

The law of similars was observed to operate by Hahnemann and others before him rather like we observe the law of gravity to operate – these are empirical laws.

From the proving we have a picture of the symptoms a drug can produce. We know that the true dynamic inner disease (Central Disturbance) expresses itself in the totality of symptoms. The Law of Similars says if the drug picture is similar to the patient's symptom picture this drug will surely cure.

> *...and, moreover, the totality of these its symptoms, ...must be the principal, or the sole means, whereby the disease can make known what remedy it requires – the only thing that can determine the choice of the most appropriate remedy – and thus, in a word, the totality of the symptoms must be the principal, indeed the only thing the physician has to take note of in every case of disease and to remove by means of his art, in order that the disease shall be cured and transformed into health.*

> *(Stanza 7)*

2.8 ENHANCING SYMPTOMS

Since the symptoms of disease are beneficial to the individual as a whole, we seek to enhance or strengthen these symptoms. Therefore we give a medicinal substance (in an appropriate potency, dose and frequency) which, known to create similar symptoms in the healthy, will surely strengthen the existing symptom picture of the patient thus lending sufficient strength to the Vital Force to overcome the true internal source of the disease (the Central Disturbance). The vitality now becomes strong enough to restore health to a level where disease symptoms are no longer required to manifest and cure ensues. Clearly we must aim to cure the Central Disturbance which is the true seat of the disease and this will cure all the manifestations of the disease on every level.

Throughout the application of the Law of Similars, of provings and when observing patients' symptom pictures the principle of treating the unique nature of each individual and the principle of treating them as a whole (on all our four levels) must apply.

2.9 SUPPRESSION

Suppression is the deliberate attempt to remove symptoms regardless of their true inner cause or the greater needs of the person as a whole. The Peripheral Disturbance is removed but the Central Disturbance which is causing it is untouched (refer to Diagram 6).

If the causal factor remains, it will produce symptoms again, either the same symptoms or, if the treatment has been detrimental, even worse (inner) symptoms and a new more harmful local disease picture results. Conventional medical thinking sees as unconnected these sequences of disease and fails to comprehend the true needs of the patient.

It is clear that any method of treatment is capable of removing the local disease if this is the intention. If the needs of the whole person are neglected, when for example, treating an eczema with cortisone cream, reflexology, herbal creams or homœopathic medicines all these can suppress the symptoms to the detriment of the whole person.

The only correct treatment is to treat the totality of symptoms – including mental and emotional symptoms, also taking into account causation, concomitants and to give proper regard to the correct grading of importance of all these symptoms – in the light of our knowledge of the true causes of disease.

Suppression of disease requires the intention to suppress, that is to persist in the treatment until the symptoms disappear or mutate. Merely choosing a less than perfect remedy will not be suppressive; it will not cure fully but there remains the opportunity to re-assess the case; and select a more similar remedy. Repeated wrong prescribing may confuse or distort the symptom totality and thereby spoiling the case; so restraint does need to be exercised in intractable cases. Diagram 6 illustrates that if we aim our treatment at the Peripheral Disturbance (PD) and neglect the cause of the disease, which is in the Central Disturbance, we are in danger of suppressing the disease and reducing the patient's health.

ENLIGHTENED SUPPRESSION In fact we frequently suppress symptoms when we prescribe. If the true needs of the patient are not perceived, if the real deep cause of the disease is not treated, yet the symptoms are ameliorated, then this is suppression. It may be necessary to prescribe this kind of 'enlightened' suppression as a short term measure because the patient is only able to take one step at a time towards cure . The prescriber's intention is not to be satisfied with suppression but merely to postpone deeper cure. The prescriber's own depth and range of awareness in deciding what is to be cured also decides at what level to cure. The Organon aims at "the highest ideal of cure", but each one of us has a different ideal, and each patient also has a different level of cure with which they are satisfied.

2.10 PRINCIPLES IX AND X

We have now added two further principles of practice:

PRINCIPLE IX
The principle of using potentised remedies.

---

and

PRINCIPLE X
The principle of similars, to enhance patient symptoms so as to strengthen the action of the vital force.

We now have a truly scientific method of healing. We know precisely what each of our medicines will do in detail from provings. When we elicit the full and accurate symptom picture, of the patient and match this with as similar as possible a drug picture cure will be inevitable. However, Stanza 3 warns us that there may be further obstacles to cure and that the Physician must know what these are and how to remove them.

if he finally knows the obstacles to recovery in each case and is aware of how to remove them, so that the restoration of health may be permanant ...

(Stanza 3)

The original causes of chronic disease and of susceptibility have to be known and removed. In Chapter 4 we take up this subject of the causes of disease in more depth.

EXERCISES

1. Define susceptibility in the context of becoming ill.
2. Use the concept of susceptibility to analyse a) the impact of vaccination on people and b) to discuss why virulent plagues and epidemics do not wipe out the entire population.
3. Define AIDS and discuss what you know about this disease in terms of immunity and suscepibility.
4. You can remove the symptoms of a disease in two ways, either by making the patient more healthy, or paradoxically, by making them more sick. Explain this paradox.

RECOMMENDED READING FOR CHAPTER II

Close, Stuart 'The Genius of Homœopathy' Chapter 13

Hahnemann, Samuel 'The Organon of Medicine' Stanzas 3, 5, 7, 21-27, 34,
    46-51,61, 70-71, 82, 104, 146-154, 186, 201, 225, 261

Kent, James Tyler 'Lectures on Homœopathic Philosophy' Chapter 5

Roberts, Herbert 'The Principles, Art and Science of Homœopathy'
    Chapters 4, 6, 7, 8, 13

Shepherd, Dorothy 'Homœopathy in Epidemic Diseases'

Vithoulkas, George 'The Science of Homœopathy'
    Chapters 1, 2, 4, 5, 9, 10, 11, 14

Wright Hubbard, Elizabeth 'A Brief Study Course in Homœopathy'
    Chapters 7,14

Chapter III

A PROFILE OF THE PATIENT

1. The Hierarchy of Symptoms
2. The Totality of Symptoms and Beyond
3. Delusions, Dreams and Fears.
4. Taking the Case – The First Homœopathic Interview.
5. Introduction to the Repertory.
6. Notes
   > Casetaking Checklist
   > Anatomical Order of Rubrics
7. Exercises
8. Recommended Reading

3.1 THE HIERARCHY OF SYMPTOMS

We are going to look here at the relative importance of symptoms, also known as the hierarchy of symptoms, and its importance in deciding what is to be cured. From The Organon we read:

From this indubitable truth, that besides the totality of the symptoms, with considerations of the accompanying modalities, nothing can by any means be discovered in diseases wherewith they could express their need of aid, it follows undeniably that the sum of all the symptoms and conditions in each individual case of disease must be the sole indication, the sole guide to direct us in the choice of a remedy.

(Stanza 18) (Read again Stanza 7 also)

We learn from these Stanzas that the totality of symptoms gives us the accurate picture of the whole disease. Not all symptoms are of equal value. Some symptoms are the result of deeper, more powerful and more essential causes than others. We have described how negative thought patterns produce symptoms in the lower levels of the being and we have noted that powerful emotions also bring about changes on the physical level (I.6). Observation of symptoms must take account of:

1. The location in the hierarchy of the organism. For example a cut on the chest is less serious than a cut on the heart.
2. The intensity of the symptom in the patient – how strong is it?
3. The degree of peculiarity of the symptom. Symptoms which reflect the uniqueness of the individual are called characteristic symptoms. They are important because they reflect the inner states of the person. These symptoms are also called keynote symptoms and they may be strange, rare or even peculiar.

The quality of a symptom is most important, the symptoms that reflect unique individual needs and unique individual reactions are most valuable.

PRINCIPLE XI
The principle of the hierarchical nature of symptoms and its correspondence to the hierarchy found in the natural universe.

3.2 TOTALITY AND BEYOND

We must observe what is inner, causative and deepest in our patients if we are to correctly grade the symptoms and cure the inner state or the Central Disturbance. This Central State which when disturbed brings about illness in an individual is called also the 'essence of the person'. Hahnemann calls this essence the 'disposition' of the patient.

> *... and in all cases of disease we are called on to cure, the state of the patient's disposition is to be particularly noted, along with the totality of the symptoms, if we would trace an accurate picture of the disease, in order to be able therefore to treat it homœopathically with success.*
>
> *(Stanza 210)*

> *This holds good to such an extent, that the state of the disposition of the patient often chiefly determines the selection of the homœopathic remedy, as being a decidedly characteristic symptom which can least of all remain concealed from the accurately observing physician.*
>
> *(Stanza 211)*

The most skillful art the homœopath must aquire is receiving the case. The first homœopathic interview is of the utmost importance. Stanza 1 notes that it is the "physician's only calling to cure"; to not in any way become attached to your patient. A caring compassionate detachment is essential. The qualities of a good interviewer are to be able to observe and to listen. To do both these things you must have a completely still mind.

The unprejudiced observer – well aware of the futility of tran-scendental speculations which can receive no confirmation from experience – be his powers of penetration ever so great, takes note of nothing in every individual disease, except the changes in the health of the body and of the mind (morbid phenomena, accidents, symptoms) which can be perceived externally by means of the senses; that is to say, he notices only the deviations from the former healthy state of the now dis-eased individual, which are felt by the patient himself, remarked by those around him and observed by the physician. All these perceptible signs represent the disease in its whole extent, that is, together they form the true and only conceivable portrait of the disease.

(Stanza 6)

The most important symptoms are mental and emotional. I want now to intro-duce you to a world of fantasy, the surreal and the archetype, to the world of film and fiction, to the world of delusion, dreams and fears. These worlds contain the inner symptoms that the patient will show and describe. These deep symptoms will however be couched in the terms of the everyday, the mundane and familiar. These symptoms are there to see and understand, they are not hidden in dark secrecy but expressed freely in everyday lan-guage and gesture for the detailed observer free from prejudice to see.

3.3 DELUSIONS DREAMS AND FEARS

A delusion is a sensation or thought which is not warranted by the facts. Everyone has some delusions, which may not be obvious, but manifest themselves as a fixed idea or a prejudice. An illusion is similar in that it is a false impression but it is known by the patient to be false, whilst an hallucina-tion is a false impression thought by the patient to be real. In many cases delusions are held without the patient being aware of their influence. A delu-sion may be a simple one, for example, that all members of a certain class are insensitive in some way, or that it is very difficult to get a good job if you have not been to university, or that everyone is judging you, etc. Some of these delusions make up such characteristic ideas of a person so as to be typical of them. These key symptoms or delusions can make up the essence of the remedy picture. For example a person may be afraid of meeting anybody new or of undertaking anything new for fear of failure, the key idea being the delusion that they are too weak mentally and physically to stand the strain of the encounter or of the new task. All symptoms stem from this delusion, the body's muscles will become weak and the assimilation of food faulty in a physical reflection of the mental symptom. The whole person on every level suffers a lack of confidence and an inability to complete things. Physically, stools are 'bashful', splinters fester and fail to be expelled, etc. You may recognise symptoms of the homœopathic remedy *Silica*.

Delusions can stem from childhood conditioning, "my father always criticised me and I was told constantly that I was useless". In due course this person becomes *Anarcardium* and must battle constantly with his inferiority complex to say "I am OK, I can do it".

A delusion may come from an accident, a shock, a fear or from any experience including a natural disaster or war.

A delusion may also be held because it has been ingrained into the subconscious at conception, 'in utero' or even from the influence of one's forbears.

The subconscious is the true home of our delusions, which are deep beliefs colouring our every thought, reaction and act. The subconscious also makes itself known to us in our sleep. Dreams will often give us a clue to the delusions we are labouring under. Our fears will also reflect a cause forgotten, remote or ancestral which has given us an emotional or mental stance that colours our every thought and action.

This is the place in which we find our true inner symptoms, the causal essences which make us what we are.

3.4 TAKING THE CASE – THE FIRST INTERVIEW

The essential needs for taking the case are:

1. An appropriate environment, pleasant, private and friendly.
2. An attitude of compassionate detachment; if a patient cries, for example, then pause, offer a handkerchief, wait and gently proceed. You need to establish a good contact.
3. The aim of case taking is to dIscover what is to be cured. Observe and listen, do not ask lots of questions. Begin by asking "How can I help you?" this is positive and open ended. You should already have some preliminary information, perhaps from a sheet the patient completes before arriving at the clinic. When the patient has given you the details of their complaints then ask, "is there anything else?"– and go on asking this until they have told you everything.
4. Do not hurry, give the patient the chance to answer from their depths.
5. Observe and assess what you observe. There is rarely a need to ask questions about every area of the human condition (see the notes to this chapter). You do need to ask the questions which are relevant to the patient which you have discerned from a) observing them, and b) what their troubles are and how they relate to them.
6. You must know the following secret. The patient tells you the most important things without realising it and at a moment when they are not directly answering your questions. Be on guard for the things that reveal the 'delusion' which reveals the essence of their case.
7. Now you are prepared to gently prompt the patient to give you their secrets. After you have noted the details of the presenting complaint, then determine the patient's highest symptoms, the mental and emotional. The patients demeanour, gestures, manner and the nature of the presenting complaint should give you a guide as to the type of person and therefore the areas of importance which your case taking should explore.
8. Additionally, it is necessary to explore certain important areas
    –   The emotional reaction – is the patient open or closed?

- The existence of anticipatory fears, other fears or phobias.
- The reaction to personal loss and the ability to grieve.
- The ability to weep.
- The degree of tidiness or fastidiousness.
- The presence of strong emotions – and how they are expressed.
- The quality of their mental faculties.
- Dreams.
- Is the patient trusting or suspicious?
- How easily can the patient give and receive?
- The nature of their temper. Is it quick, slow, forgotten easily?
- Do they sulk, bear grudges, forgive or not?
- Are they hurried, impetuous or careful?
- Sexual expression.

After this, the essence of the case should be narrowed down and differential diagnosis is possible by confirming or rejecting particular remedies. Now you can refer to:

9. Physical Generals, as expressed in:
   - Temperature, weather, covering and perspiration.
   - Sleep and the effects of sleep. Good and bad times of the day.
   - Appetite, tastes, digestion. Bowel and bladder functions.
   - The effect of movement, pressure and touch.
   - The menstrual cycle in all its aspects, sexual expression, contraception past and present, childbirth experience.

10. In the course of the interview construct a chronological time line of everything that has happened to the patient from conception to the present moment. This time line of life events must begin with inheritance; take a careful record of family medical history including as many generations as is known of. Include uncles, aunts, cousins, nephews, nieces, and the patient's own children. You will usually have to probe. Few patients fail to hide away some of the disease tendencies they are heir to. Inquire into the presence of miasms (see Chapter 4).

11. Childhood experience and the full nature of the patient as a child is of the utmost importance.

12. Ascertain if there have been any big disappointments, frights, shocks, etc as well as any physical trauma. It is important to know the patient's detailed reaction at the time of impact of all these things. Given the same trauma different people will react differently. You must know the facts of each case.

3.4 (II) HINTS ON HOW TO QUESTION THE PATIENT

To obtain this information you must ask questions and observe the patient's reaction, in doing this note the following:

1. Ask only general open-ended questions, for example, not, "Are you jealous?" but, "What is the strongest emotion you feel most frequently?". If in the presenting complaint a hint of a suppressed emotion is given you may ask questions like, "What is your reaction to someone who is rude or unfair to you?" etc. This type of question is less likley to bias the answer.

2. Ask for specific examples, for instance, "When did you last cry?", "When did you last lose your temper", etc. Homœopathic cure must be based on facts and it must be scientific. It can only be based on facts if we can discern them.

3. Every symptom must be traced to its origin. If you are told that the patient finds it difficult to tolerate criticism, you must ask "Why?". "Why?" to every answer until you reach the essential 'cause' or 'delusion' which results in a particular symptom.

4. You must not accept any qualitative answer on its face value. For example, "Are you thirsty?" is a direct question of little value. "Yes" could mean anything. We want to know:
   - Does the patient feel dryness; where and how severely?
   - How often does the patient take a drink?
   - How big is the cup?
   - How much do they drink of each cup?
   - How do they drink it, ie quickly or in sips?

We must have the facts. If you ask, "How is your feeling for sex?" and the patient responds, "Normal", what does this mean? To one person normal is coition once a month, and to another it may be three times a day.

If a child loses his temper find out how much and to what effect. Note that parents will often underestimate the bad side and exaggerate the good side of their children's behaviour. Probe into all areas until you have all the facts and the ultimate causes.

It can be useful to quantify qualities by putting them on a scale of 1-10 or expressing them as a percentage. This becomes meaningful when there are changes over a period of time. For example, the severity of a pain may improve by 30% in one month.

3.4 (III) ASSESSMENT

When you have all the information from a patient as to Essence, Totality and Keynotes, there should form a clear pattern of a remedy picture. Now look to see that this picture truly matches the person sitting before you. Also observe if there are any, even slight, contradictions in the case information. Any contradiction means you have not completed the symptoms fully, you have not found the true symptoms or motive or 'delusion' which informs this area of the patient's behaviour. For example, you may note that a patient is emotionally closed yet that they enjoy consolation and sympathy. The closed patient usually prefers to be alone in moments of grief or sadness. What is the real picture?

It is necessary to complete every symptom as to modality, causation, concomitant and thus discover its origin – in its origin you will find the Essence.

In the notes to this chapter you will find a comprehensive list of points to inquire into when taking the case. This list represents a laborious, time-consuming task but you are advised to use this and go through it (or a similar one) when you first begin to practice taking the case on your family and friends. Make a shorter checklist to keep by you when interviewing. At first it will be hard to see the wood for the trees. However, remember the important principles and seek the highest symptoms, the essential blockage to the creativity of the patient, and what is 'applicable' to each individual case. As you become more skilled in these areas case-taking will become more immediate and effective.

> *This individualising examination of the case, for which I shall only give in this place general directions, of which the practitioner will bear in mind only what is applicable for each individual case, demands of the physician nothing but freedom from prejudice and sound senses, attention in observing and fidelity in tracing the picture of the disease.*
>
> *(Stanza 83)*

3.5 INTRODUCTION TO REPERTORY WORK

Look at "Kent's Repertory to the Materia Medica". You will see a bewildering array of symptoms, called Rubrics, with remedies listed under these rubrics.

The Repertory confuses and misleads more often than it helps. There are several mistakes the novice makes in using the Repertory, these are to consult the Repertory:

1. Before all the symptoms have been found.
2. Before you have graded all the symptoms and established a hierarchy of depth of symptoms.
3. Before you have studied the chronology of symptoms and life events of the patient and assessed this with reference to the grading of importance.
4. Before you have completed every symptom to discover the true essence, delusion or cause and therefore the correct rubric to use in the repertory.

Repertorising the wrong symptoms will produce a convincingly wrong remedy and this will be especially comforting if it is produced on a computer display screen. It is best to take the case completely so you need only repertorise a few crucial, essential symptoms.

TYPE VARIATION

Kent's Repertory uses a system of black type, italic and low type remedies. These refer to the number of people who experienced this symptom in the provings. In practice this is not only a quantitive measure, it is also a good indication of the intensity of the symptom.

Unless otherwise indicated, a rubric entry means that the patient is aggravated, eg. look up under Generalities on page 1357, "Eating while" means there is general aggravation while eating. On page 1349, "heat and cold" means the patient is aggravated by both.

The Mind section covers both mental and emotional symptoms. Generalities includes a lot of pathology, and also causes, like injuries. Under the Stomach section you will find desires and aversions, but when a food or drink aggravates, you will find this in Generalities under Food.

For any symptom we need to know:
What it feels like? = Sensation
Where is it? = Location
Does it move anywhere? = Extension
What affects or changes it and how? = Modality
What caused it? – if known – this can be obvious or
subtle, physical, emotional or intellectual = Causation
What else is happening at the same time
in other parts of the patient? = Concomitants

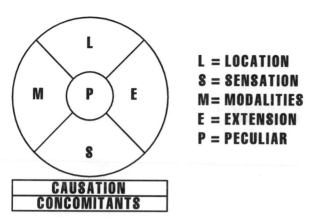

L = LOCATION
S = SENSATION
M = MODALITIES
E = EXTENSION
P = PECULIAR

Diagram 7

Chapter 3 notes

CASETAKING CHECKLIST

Checklist of areas to enquire into when taking the case:

DAILY HABITS

- daily routine including sleep, cleanliness, exercise, food and drink taken daily etc
- smoking, tea, coffee, drugs, alcohol

PERSONAL
- ask about own birth – ie normal, breech, induced, Caesarean
- ask if breastfed and for how long
- vaccinations – type, quantity, sequence and reaction to them
- childhood complaints – measles, chicken pox, German measles, mumps, whooping cough, scarlet fever, impetigo; or if any other illnesses find out the sequence if possible. Find out severity and if any residues or after-effects
- ask if any accidents and look for any residues
- ask if any operations or shocks which took a while to get over
- also if they have had epilepsy, petit mal, skin complaints, warts, verrucas, glandular fever (mononucleosis), hay fever, asthma.

Ask patient if he dates any of his present complaints from past illnesses, vaccinations, accidents etc.

FAMILY
- find out the main possible hereditary factors in the family tree ie parents, grandparents and especially uncles and aunts: what did they die of or

suffer from. Look in particular for TB, asthma, hayfever, cancer (syphilis, gonorrhoea).

Note – general appearance – age, build, colouring, posture (how stand and sit), manner (restless, despondent, happy etc), dress, set and colour of eyes, hair, face (colour,expression etc), voice (quality, production, vocabulary), body odour. General constitution.

Observe and note – how the mind of the patient works; patient's reaction to the prescriber, to the world in general. Attitude to life. This is amongst the most important information, that which is observed by the prescriber but is not freely given by the patient. Receiving this information becomes easier with knowledge of the Materia Medica, people and practice. It is an interesting exercise to sit in a public place and spot the remedies.

Observe the patient's reaction to his condition, how it affects him. You may have to dig for it, however it is pure gold if you can find it.

PHYSICAL

Vertigo – note modalities etc, how it started and aftermath. If the room is seen to go round or if it is in the head and the room remains still. Tendency to fall, which way? Any ear trouble as concomitant, pains etc. Nausea. The use of alcohol can often < or mitigate vertigo, also loss of sleep.

Head – in general
Headaches – location and extension, sensation (includes type of pain), modalities
Eyes and vision
Ears and hearing and reaction to noise (if deafness, find out if < wandering attention or not wanting to hear something)
Nose and smell
Catarrh – colour, modalities, history etc
Mouth and taste, including gums (bleeding, swollen, sore etc), teeth, tongue, ulcers etc.

Throat – sore, or ulcers, or difficulty swallowing, pains, constrictions,or sense of a lump or a band etc.

Digestive system – nausea, vomiting, eructations, flatulence, constipation, and diarrhoea. If stool loose, lumpy, hard, dry. If with wind, blood, mucous or any pains or sensations.

Appetite – important to note what they feel like eating rather than what they think they should eat. A lot of people are faddish about food.
–   How feel before, during, after meal.
–   What are the results of fasting or missing a meal. When is hunger experienced – night?
–   If hungry and hunger vanishes after a few bites, if have trouble afterwards and if this trouble is soon after or a few hours after.
–   What kinds of food make them sick – sour, greasy, eggs, meat, pork, bread, butter, vegetables, onions (boiled), cabbage, fruit, wine, beer, coffee, tea, milk, vinegar, spirits.
–   For what foods do they a have marked craving or what kinds of drinks (same list as for <s)
–   How much salt do they use (if add before tasting), also pepper, mustard, pickles, sauce.
–   How much sugar – in tea, puddings, etc.
–   How many sweets in a day (Mars bars, etc)
–   Find out if they crave any foods which then < (ie if they react badly to something they like).

Abdomen – check for pains, sensitivities etc, in liver, spleen, kidneys, intestines, angles of colon etc.

Rectum – check for haemorrhoids, fissures, bleedings, itchings, oozings, pains etc.

Urination – any difficulties, pain, discomforts, check for frequency and times, deposits, cloudy, hot, if urination >s or <s, general changes in its nature, including odour.

Sexual Expression

This is related to the whole person and requires special care and attention. The ease or difficulty students and practitioners have in enquiring about and understanding the relative importance of a patient's sexual expression reflects the questioner's own freedom or restiction in this area. Our sexual expression is intimately related to the essence of our being and often gives the key to our Central Disturbance. Some homœopaths gloss over sexual symptoms through fear of embarrasing or antagonising the patient and, thus the deeper needs of the patient are not met.

I suggest that the difficulties which homœopaths have around sex stem from a confusion about what is pathological and what is normal or healthy. We are aiming to give expression to the 'higher purposes' of our 'indwelling reason gifted mind'. How then are our higher purposes served by sex? Is our eternal spirit interested in whether we masturbate? If we enjoy sex with the same or opposite gender? If we like sex with two partners? If we indulge in adventurous variations with our complying lover? I would suggest that what causes disease is none of these things but the confusion, guilt and other negative feelings created in our emotional vehicle by the failure to be honest about our needs.

It is also necessary to enquire on the physical side of:
– any discharges, disabilities, history of VD, perversions of desire, ie masturbation, homosexuality, etc.

Menstrual History

– Age periods began (12-14 is normal), if troublesome.
– Frequency, regularity.
– If painful, nature of pain, modalities, etc esp. if <heat or cold and if >hot water bottle or stretching out.
– Duration, abundance, colouring, odour, clots.

- When is flow greatest and least
- How does she feel before, during and after menses
- Any other discharges at any other time – character ie colour, odour, consistency, modalities, if irritates or stains.
- If on 'Pill' – how long, what effect. Any other effect of contraceptive methods.

General sex– if hyper or hypo; or feelings absent, or perverted. Any homosexual desires or activities.

Also check if any operations or treatment (esp. hormones); check for hysterectomy; if tubes cut; or if had problems at menopause.

Respiration and Cough – if wheezy breathing; moist or dry; rattling and if <climbing stairs; if <hot/dry or cold/wet or any change; cough – if <hot air, cold air, hot-cold-hot, or any changes or times. Nature of cough, nature of discharge, if any; intervals; if affects any other part, which one and how. What affects the cough – eg. eating, drinking, laughing. If any hayfever, colds, coryza, asthma or nervous asthma, air hunger.

Chest, Lungs and Heart – chest – describe pain – burning, stabbing, throbbing, catching etc if <breathing (in and/or out)
Lungs – find out which region affected
Heart – check thoroughly (NB varicose veins, prolapse, piles and hernia are all linked with heart trouble). Look for palpitations, anginas, tachycardia, pain down left/right arm. Breathlessness, from exercise, climbing stairs. Note if there is any pain felt in arm on taking BP or pulse; if so, heart trouble is imminent.
Pulse – take more than 30, note its nature.
Blood pressure – take BP to establish an average.
Back – check for pains, aches, sore spots, disabilities etc, if pains, find where, when, what <s and >s.

Neck – (trouble at top of spine/base of skull should be put with head).

Extremities – the largest section in the Repertory

Circulation – cold hands and feet; blueness and other changes of colour; hot or cold flushes; arms and legs go to sleep.

Nervous system – loss of power or paralysis; tremors or spasms with pains and modalities; numbness or oversensitivity; general nervous condition.

Skin – any eruptions – get full description, eg. scaly, pointed, messy, single, groups, etc, what kind of discharge – watery, gummy, purulent, oily, etc; periodicity, time of year, situation in life – ie exams, meetings etc or if <too much make-up or frustrations, or from not washing. Also its location. Note if ulcerations, if itching – <heat or cold or from uncovering regardless of heat or cold, <scratching or >scratching or <water, etc.

Sleep and dreams
– Find out if sleep in any particular position – ie on stomach, or knee-chin position, or arms over head, or with legs spread wide, or on one side or the other etc.
– How many pillows (ie if head held high).
– If they have been told that they talk, laugh, shriek or walk in their sleep.
– What time do they go to sleep – how easily, when do they wake up, dothey go back to sleep easily, what disturbs them, if they wake in the night do they get up; if no, what do they do.
– If can't sleep – from mind full of ideas, ie overactive, or from something on the mind, one idea eg. resentment, fear, conscience.
– Do they dream – find out if related to digestion or if from threatening conditions (sepsis/toxicity) or if haunting dreams (rewrite dream) or if recurring dream.
Fever – chill, heat, sweat.
   Note – chill during sweat; dry during heat; no sweat; or does sweat >?

Check extent of sweat and any abnormalities; if inadequate sweat – check other secretions. If thirsty with chill, if thirsty with sweat, heat etc.

Generals and Modalities

Seasons – if has hayfever etc find out which season. Look also for spring or autumn <s or < or > in any season.

Weather – what sort of weather do they dislike most, ie cold, damp, or dry, cold, or fog or snow or sunny etc.

How do they feel when the weather changes?

If <before, during or after a storm. (If <thunderstorms and are <before, will usually be tense people; If <during, look for more nervous habits, fears; If <after, need outlet for their life force, (are dammed up).

Reaction to wind – if N, S, E, W or wind in general.

Which climate would they choose to live in?

Temperature – find out about warmth in general – warmth of bed, of room, of fire, find out about draughts in air; changes in temperature, extremes of temperature.

How do they dress in winter?

If keep window open at night.

How does sea bathing affect them?

How do they react to cold or hot baths?

Position and motion – Find out position liked best or which gives most relief; eg. if >bending double, stretching backwards, standing up, lying down or on feet if moving but <if standing around.

If pain < or >continued movement. If <limbering up, after moving for some time, when resting again.

If move in bed, find out if because movement >pain or if bed hard or uncomfortable.

If don't move in bed find out if because movement <pain or pain >by lying still or lying on painful side or other side etc.

How do they react to standing for a while or kneeling.

Pressure – if < or >touch, or if <light touch >pressure or if <firm grip and >light touch.

Locality/Sidedness – find out if complaints or pains are limited to one side or locality, eg. left-sided complaints or right-sided, or right arm left leg, or left arm and right leg, or right upper half and left lower half etc.

Times – find out if complaint or person are worse or better at any particular time or times eg. <3am or 4-8pm or <on waking or <evenings, <night or >night, >3pm or >after sleep etc.

General – reaction to heights, how do they feel at the seaside or the mountains, when do they feel like fainting, reaction to tight collars, belts or tight clothing etc. (NB try not to ask direct questions).

Sensations – if have any unusual sensations

– sensation as if – eg. lump in the throat (which may or may not be 'real'),

eg. worms or a tumour or just a sensation.

– real – (are a good indication) the more unusual the better.

NBWS – look for any 'never been well since...' symptoms. They can be very important.

MENTAL AND EMOTIONAL

Seek always for the outstanding or unusual or recently changed symptoms since some mental symptoms are always present.

The following are only suggested questions. Each of you must develop your own way of 'receiving' the information.

– When during your day would you feel sad, or depressed or pessimistic? Then enquire if the sadness ever becomes despair/despondency?

– How do worries affect you? Do you have any particular worries at the moment?

– On what sort of occasion would you weep?

– How do you tolerate consolation or fuss?

– How do you like being alone?

– How do you feel in a roomful of people – eg. parties, lectures, meetings etc?

– How do you feel about having to entertain people?

– What sort of thing would make you anxious or even fearful?

If no certain reply ask about – animals, burglars, falling, heights, water, being alone, loss of reason or insanity, night, darkness, the future, being ill, poverty, certain diseases (cancer, TB, syphilis etc).

- Under what conditions would you become angry, or what makes you angry? (What do you do with your anger?)
- How do you tolerate waiting?
- Do other people say you walk, talk, eat or write quickly?
- When you're depressed how do you look at death -(sus presentiment of, desire for, check also tendency to suicide).
- When would you feel jealous? (check how deeply/strongly).
- Some people are tidy and others are not so tidy – how do you see yourself?
- Have you ever had any deep shocks of an emotional nature – how did it affect you? (Note what it was and its effects).
- How much do your periods affect your emotions or mind?
- How do you tolerate contradiction?
- Under what conditions would you feel confused?
- Some people are suspicious and others aren't – how do you see yourself?
- Do you tend to contradict others?
- When would you be critical?
- How are you about making decisions? Do you stick to your decisions?
- How is your concentration?
- Are you easily startled?
- Some people are reserved or quiet and others are extroverted, how are you?
- What kind of people do you admire?
- How is your memory? – (sus what is the exact problem).
- How is your sense of time and distance?
- Some people are always optimistic and others sometimes feel they are incurable – how do you see yourself? – or how do other people see you?
- What type of fantasies or imaginations do you have?

- People have various attitudes to money – how are you about money matters?
- How much are you affected by grief, fright, love, indignation, disappointment, vexation?

PAIN

If the patient has pain, use these questions to fill out your symptom picture: (NB do not just add it on after mental/emotional questions).
- What time of day of night is it worse or better?
- What is its exact position?
- When do they notice the pain move to another part of the body?
- When do they get relief from pain?
- What sort of weather makes it worse?
- What do they notice about the pain when the weather changes, say dry to wet or vice-versa.
- How does warmth affect it (general or of arm, leg etc)?
- How does movement affect it (general or of arm, leg etc)?
- How does pressure affect it (eg hair, clothes, lying on it or loosening clothes etc)?
- How does rubbing affect the painful part?
- Find out any other modalities which affect it or the person.

Sometimes pathological diagnostic symptoms are found as a sub heading under the place involved, eg pleurisy as 'Chest, inflammation, pleura, of'; or appendicitis as 'Abdomen, inflammation, appendicitis', etc.

Objective symptoms are scattered all through the Repertory and often small, unclassified rubrics such as 'Gestures' under Mind or 'Cling' under Mind, 'red lips' under 'Face, discolouration, red, lips of', etc.

There are no sections for the circulatory, glandular or nervous system but the parts of these symptoms are found scattered throughout the Repertory under the appropriate anatomical heading. Many nervous symptoms appear in Generalities such as analgesia, chorea, convulsions, paralysis, trembling, etc. Twitching of parts appears in the section dealing with those.

Pain where it affects the whole person is under Generalities. Where it involves parts see under that part.In general pain is laid out as follows:

Pain – generally in regard to tissue, and other conditions (alphabetic) then; Pain – localised in regard to time, other condition; extension, then; Character of pain generally, time, other condition, extension, then; Character of pain in regard to each locality in turn – time, conditions, extension.

EXERCISES

1. On what way are people affected by an epidemic who are suffering from
   (a) mild chronic disease?
   (b) grave chronic disease?
2. What exactly do you understand by unprejudiced observation? What are the most common elements which prevent a Homœopath from achieving the ability to be an unprejudiced observer?
3. From memory make a list of the questions you would ask in taking the case. Then go over the list and see how many questions were in any way leading or direct. How would you change these to help them give you more symptoms which were unique or characteristic to the patient?
4. If you were allowed only twenty questions to ask when taking the case which twenty would you select.
5. Prepare a brief checklist to summarise your case taking questionnaire and procedure which you can keep by you.
6. Give examples of symptoms and how to complete them or take them to their ultimate origin.
7. Place the correct page number of the relevant rubric in Kent's Repertory in the brackets below.

ANATOMICAL ORDER OF RUBRICS

Mind (   ) includes sensitive to light, noise etc but not smell
which is in Nose.

Vertigo (   ) levitation, sinking, falling to R or L.

Head (   ) includes hair, meningitis – as Head, inflammation, meninges, of.
– also see Back

Eyes (   ) and Vision (   )

Ears (   ) and Hearing (   )

Nose (   ) includes some sinuses, and sense of Smell (   )

Face (   ) includes salivary glands, some sinuses, lips.

Mouth (   ) includes tongue – (under mouth discolouration)
and speech, also in Mind (   ).

Throat (   ) includes cervical glands, thyroid, goitre

NB Back contains posterior neck and nape.

Stomach (   ) includes oesophagus (has some Generals – desires
and aversions in regard to diet and hunger and thirst.

NB better or worse for eating and drinking and for different foods are found in
Generalities.

Abdomen (   ) includes liver, (most of the menstrual pains – if you can't differentiate between gastric and abdominal pain consult both sections).
Includes appendicitis as 'inflammation, appendicitis'.

Rectum (   ) diarrhoea, constipation, urging are found under Rectum,
whereas character of Stool has its own section (   ).

Urinary organs (   ) has five sections: Bladder (   ), urging, retention, etc
Kidneys (   ). Prostate (   ). Urethra (   ). Urine (   ).includes character
of urine and copious or scanty.

Genitalia (   ) has two sections, Male (   ) and Female (   )under Female
are some generalities associated with menses but general modalities related
to menses are under Generalities (includes type and circumstance, in particular of menses). Mental states affected by menses – see under Mind; also
some in Abdomen.

'Menses' as a modality is found in all sections.

Larynx and trachea (   ) voice is included.

Respiration (   )

Cough (   ) and Expectoration (   )

Chest (   ) includes lungs, heart, mammae, mild, axillary glands, aorta.

Pleurisy – as 'chest, inflammation, pleura, of, emphysema

Back (   ) includes posterior neck, nape, cervical region, nervous symptoms related to the spine appear here.

Meningitis – see Head.

Extremities (   )

Sleep (   ) includes Dreams, includes position.

NB 'better or worse for sleep' and for different positions lying are gesia, chorea, convulsions, paralysis, trembling, etc Twitching of parts appears in the section dealing with those.

Pain where it affects the whole person is under Generalities. Where it involves parts see under that part.In general pain is laid out as follows:

Pain – generally in regard to tissue, and other conditions (alphabetic) then; Pain – localised in regard to time, other condition; extension, then; Character of pain generally, time, other condition, extension, then; Character of pain in regard to each locality in turn – time, conditions, extension. under Generalities.

Chill (   )

Fever (   ) includes the succession of stages

Perspiration (   ) for 'better or worse from perspiration' as a whole see under Genaralities. This section includes quality, occurrence and modality of discharge itself. Sweat in any particular location will be found in that anatomical section.

Skin (   ) NB Skin only a particular, an eliminatory organ.

Generalities (   ) In this section are found the pathological or diagnostic rubrics such as measles, sycosis, scarlet fever, septicaemia, syphilis. Certain pathological states which are symptoms rather than disease are found here, eg chorea, convulsions, cyanosis, dropsy, etc

RECOMMENDED READING FOR CHAPTER 3

Bender, P 'The Examination of The Patient' B Jain Publishers

Bidwell 'How to Take the Case' B Jain Publishers

Hahnemann, Samuel 'The Organon of Medicine' Stanzas 6-25, 83-104, 210-211

Kent, James Tyler 'Lectures on Homœopathic Philosophy' Chapters 23, 24, 25, 26, 27

Rutter, Peter 'Sex in the Forbidden Zone' Unwin Paperbacks

Roberts, Herbert 'The Principles, Art and Science of Homœopathy' Chapters 8, 9, 10, 11

Vithoulkas, George 'The Science of Homœopathy' Chapter 12

Vithoulkas, George 'A New Model of Health and Disease'

Wright Hubbard, Elizabeth 'A Brief Study Course in Homœopathy' Chapters 3, 4, 5, 6, 7

Chapter IV

OBSTACLES TO RECOVERY

1. What are Miasms?
2. Hahnemann's Three Miasms – Psora, Sycosis, Syphilis
3. Additional Miasms: Tubercular and Cancer, and others
4. Identifying Miasmatic Influences
5. Prescribing on Miasms
6. Notes

> Examples of anti-miasmatic remedies
> Case example

7. Exercises
8. Recommended Reading

4.1 WHAT ARE MIASMS?

As we saw in Chapter 2, there are immediate (exciting) causes, maintaining causes and fundamental causes of disease. The last of these, fundamental causes, forms our 'soil' or susceptibility to disease, and this will be contributed to by any miasmatic influences that are present. A miasm is any inherent weakness or tendency to disease. Conventionally, the word diathesis is used to denote the constitution or general susceptibility of the body to catch disease (Blacks Medical Dictionary). It is only in homœopathic theory that we find a clear explanation of how disease susceptibility itself arises, this is the theory of miasms. The word miasm means a mist, indicating both its dynamic and its subtle, all pervading nature. The concept of miasms reaches deep into our subconscious, there is almost a mythical feel to this idea of deep and remote causes of disease in humanity.

The miasms go back millions of years, they surface, ebb, flow and fade according to the level of consciousness of mankind in any particular age. Miasms work deeply and over long periods of time, even over several generations. They work to change us so that we become more susceptible to diseases new and old. These weaknesses in our constitution can be inherited by us and in turn passed on to our children.

> *The true natural chronic diseases are those that arise from a chronic miasm, which when left to themselves, and unchecked by the employment of those remedies that are specific for them, always go on increasing and growing worse, notwithstanding the best mental and corporal regimen, and torment the patient to the end of his life with ever aggravated sufferings.*
>
> *(Stanza 78)*

A good theory or model should enable us to predict the future course of health and of susceptibility. The theory of miasms allows us to do this and therefore teaches us how to prevent as well as to remove fundamental, or underlying causes of disease. Causes "inherited, acquired and thrust upon us" can now be fully understood.

> *We can now fulfil the last of the requirements for a "true practitioner of the healing art" "...If, finally, he knows the obstacles to recovery in each case and is aware of how to remove them, so that the restoration may be permanent"*
>
> *(Stanza 3)*

Hahnemann had observed that in some cases cures were not permanent and that some deeper causes prevented this. This led him to discover those deeper causes which were his three miasms.

4.2 HAHNEMANN'S THREE MIASMS: PSORA, SYCOSIS AND SYPHILIS

The venereal diseases (and tuberculosis) are amongst those diseases which leave deep changes in the human economy and which can be inherited. We can also acquire miasms in our own lifetime, contracting a venereal infection is an obvious example. If gonorrhoea for example is suppressed with antibiotics then a miasm, more or less active, is impressed upon the constitution. This is similarly the case with syphilis and some other serious diseases.

THE PSORIC MIASM

Psorat in Hebrew means a groove and psora is well grooved into our habits of thinking and feeling. Psora is characterised by 'under-function', slowness and dullness of mind, a lack of reaction on all levels, and an inability to think independently – all of which produces slaves to formulas, dogma, and other limitations. Psora is associated physically with the 'itch', which is the first externalising of disease onto the skin, which is the most exterior part of us. Refer to the bath tub model in Chapter 1, psora causes an imperfection or under-functioning of all the channels of elimination, leading to a tendencey to the 'overflow' diseases.

We see psora manifesting as 'blind faith', where clear reason is sacrificed, nowadays on the altar of science – the new religion. Weakened by psora, our judgement and vitality impaired, we fall victim to other diseases acquired and inherited.

THE SYCOTIC MIASM

Sycosis is the 'fig-wart' miasm, and is characterised by 'over-function', overgrowth and over-secretion. Sycosis is the mother of warts, catarrh, pus and grit, the secretions of over-active mucus membranes. When the visible skin has been 'tided up' by modern external applications the inner skin, the mucus membranes begins to express these suppressed diseases in the sycotic manner of excess. Sycosis also manifests as greed, compulsive or excessive eating, boasting and displays of ego, ostentatious behaviour and constant activity to acquire and consume. This is well expressed in the materialistic society of the modern world.

THE SYPHILITIC MIASM

The spirochaete of syphilis is a disease organism that actually destroys tissue, the syphilitic miasm reflects this in representing destruction in all its forms. The disease, and the miasm it leaves behind, are both secretive and unpredictable. The miasm has a chameleon like nature which finds a myriad of different expressions. There is destructive tissue change like necrosis and ulcers; abnormalities like dwarfism and mis-shapen, puny and deformed children, peg teeth. Other syphilitic indications include affections of the middle two fingers of either hand and children who scream night and day. There is destructive and anti-social behaviour. Relationships, businesses and family ties are all destroyed as the syphilitic miasm erupts. There is a suicidal tendency and murderous violence which is unreasoning. The true syphilitic type of person can brook no contradiction and once in power becomes a sadistic murderer and butcher like Ide Amin or Stalin. Animal experimenters and torturers fall under the influence of syphilis.

There is a parallel between these three miasms and the three roots of misery of Buddhism: These are:
1. Ignorance – which is psora.
2. Greed – which is sycosis.
3. Hatred – which is syphilis.
In Diagram 3 in Chapter 1 psora can be related to Saturn and the earth element, sycosis to Jupiter and the water element, and syphilis to Mars and the fire element. The fire of the syphilitic miasm is seen both in the creative passion of one-sided genius and in the destructive aspect of fire.

4.3 ADDITIONAL MIASMS

THE TUBERCULAR MIASM

Tuberculosis thrived in the aftermath of the Industrial Revolution. The disease leaves an inherited debility seen in a tendency to upper respiratory tract infections, allergies, hay fever and on a psychological level a seething discontent manifested in the hyperactive child and those who ceaselessly desire to travel.

THE CANCER MIASM

Cancer is an overgrowth of cells and because of this tendency to over-production is therefore essentially sycotic in nature. Two elements build cancers in the body, firstly, the suppression of the natural expression of feelings and emotions. This is often based on the second element, which is fear. We live in an age of fear. Fear is bred in our culture, family and social background as is the habit of suppressing feelings and hiding them behind a front of normality. These suppressed emotions, anxieties and fears become negative patterns of thought and feelings and eventually build cancer.

Many people who have cancer diagnosed surprise their friends because they have always appeared to be such happy people who can always be relied upon in a crisis and readily support others. "There is no justice", their friends will say. But through the inexorable workings of natural laws there is in the Universe and in the life of mankind perfect justice. All cancer is diligently earned by procrustean efforts to deceive and to deny true expression of the whole self (positive and negative) by its creators.

OTHER MIASMS

Many homœopaths observe that new diatheses are being created in the modern world by the use of antibiotics and other drugs, vaccinations and by the effects of pollution. They postulate that new miasms are arising from these sources. In addition many individuals have a depleted immune system because of their reliance on modern drug treatments.

Diseases become fashionable from time to time because of clear and good reason. Acquired miasms are only acquired because of our existing susceptibilities. New diseases like AIDS for example, appear because of the dramatically enhanced susceptibility of the individual. The functioning of our immune system is a modern way of describing the ability of the Vital Force to maintain us in the best possible state of health. We can all be said to die of immune deficiency, in the sense that the Vital Force may give death as our best health posture. However when death occurs at an early age and is brought about by unnecessary suffering it offends against humanity.

At least one homœopath predicted the coming of AIDS and other, even more destructive diseases, have also been predicted. If mankind were in a better state of health we would be immune to these new diseases. Suppressive medicine weakens our health, increases our susceptibility and drives disease into deeper levels. An awareness of miasms teaches us that these effects go very deep and last a long time.

DIATHESIS

Traditionally medicine has recognised four different types of chronic disease states which in some ways reflect the miasms. They are:

1. Lymphatic Diathesis. This refers to diseases where the glands of the body are affected. As a miasm, this relates to psora and is associated with the calcium remedies.
2. Scrofulous Diathesis. This is parallel to the tubercular miasm.
3. Uric Acid or Lithaemic Diathesis. This is the rheumatic, gouty or hydrogenous diathesis and corresponds to the sycotic miasm.
4. Dyscratic Diathesis. This relates to syphilis, or more recently, to the cancer miasm.

4.4 IDENTIFYING MIASMS

When we take a case we must be careful to map out the miasmatic influences in the patient; we note their inheritance by discovering all the illnesses that members of their family have had. We need to go back into as many generations as possible, and enquire about their uncles, aunts and cousins as well as parents and grandparents and their own children.

The psoric family will have a history of anaemia, wasting diseases, skin diseases and a general tendency to be below par and not to thrive or flourish. Although members may live to an old age they suffer from slow progressive diseases.

The sycotic family has a history of warts, verrucae and growths, heart diseases, rheumatism (a disease of excess), catarrhs, gonorrhoea, bankruptcies, terms in prison, asthma, eczema of the weeping crusty kind, discharges from every orifice and finally cancers.

The syphilitic family shows a history of violence of all kinds, suicides, lunacy, drug and alcohol abuse, hermits, eccentrics, law suits, accidents, ulcers, gangrene and amputations.

The tubercular family will have a history of tuberculosis, insanity and has well-travelled members of the family like emigrants. Many respiratory problems occur in these families eg asthma, 'weak chests', lung cancer in old age. They may be at their happiest climbing a mountain or travelling to other countries, they often have an inability to 'settle down' and have the belief that the grass may be greener on the other side.

The cancer family has a sycotic type of family history but in addition you will see lots of cancer. There is also likely to be TB somewhere in the family. The cancer miasm is sometimes thought to be a combination of two or more of the other miasms. A person with a strong cancer miasm can often be a 'very nice' person, always sacrificing themselves to others wishes and often not creating the opportunity to express their own needs.

Personal history is the second area in which we see miasms manifesting. We may often see a mixture of miasmatic indications in an individual, but when there is a dominant miasmatic influence we will see similar events to those described above in the family history.

Theoretically there are many possible combinations of miasms. We may see a strongly syphilitic inheritance on the mother's side and a strong sycotic or tubercular one on the father's side. Thus we can have psora/sycosis; psora/syphilis, or sycosis/syphilis etc.

Other miasms can manifest in individuals as 'never been well since'. This could be after almost any event in their life from conception onwards. It will include imnmunisations, suppressive drug treatments, serious illness etc In each individual case we must ascertain the impact and the response to every one of these events to identify any prominent acquired miasms.

THE MODEL OF LAYERS

As mankind becomes afflicted by more and more morbific influence, these tend to build layers of disease susceptibility. Miasms build one upon another representing a deepening of ill health. The Vital Force now seeks more and more complex means to defend us against the complexities of our present condition of ill health. Therefore increasingly when we take a case now more of our patients present a complex picture reflecting multiple layers of disease. We need more sophisticated tools now to interpret and unravel symptoms which are sometimes conflicting, sometimes minimal, sometimes profuse but in disarray and reflecting no one remedy picture. However, the principles of homœopathy and the expression of disease remain unchanged and with respect to the theory of miasms Hahnemann says:

> ....the duty of a careful apprehension of its ascertainable symptoms and characteristics is as indispensable for the homœopathic physician as it was before that discovery (of miasms) as no real cure of this or other diseases can take place without a strict particular treatment, or individualisation of each case of disease.
>
> *(Stanza 82)*

We must become skilled in recognising how and when layers have been added and in judging the impact of each one and the hierarchy of importance of each and every change. We still have to take a totality of symptoms, complete every symptom, fit each symptom into its proper place in the hierarchy of importance to the individual patient and so reveal the essence of the susceptibility and matching remedy picture. This essence reveals the patients creative process, why and how they make their world what it is and why they have the illnesses they have. This is all created by their delusions, thought patterns and emotional expression.

4.5 PRESCRIBING AND MIASMS

Mankind has changed enormously in response to the myriad of changes in the world around us over the past two hundred years. The strain on our powers to adapt has been enormous. Miasms make themselves known to us through the way our Vital Force reacts to them, which gives us symptoms.

DORMANT MIASM

Sometimes the Vital Force is able to keep the miasmatic influence quiescent. We may see in the inheritance a strong miasmatic influence and although the patient may be presenting for example, with catarrh or rheumatism other sycotic manifestations are absent. Any disease may belong to any miasm, which reinforces our first principle to individualise in every case. We cannot treat groups of people like 'sycotics' or 'syphilitics'. When a miasm is dormant we prescribe on the top layer of the totality of symptoms correctly graded ie that which is most visible at the time. The remedy which may be indicated could be any one of our many medicines.

ACTIVE MIASM

Here the Vital Force reacts to the miasm less well and is forced to produce symptoms characteristic of that miasm. For example, we may find the patient complaining of warts, catarrhs, anxieties, wandering joint pains etc, where the family and/or personal history shows a strongly sycotic picture. Here one of the many anti-miasmatic remedies such as *Thuja* or *Natrum Sulph* will be indicated but a nosode need not necessarily be given.

EXPOSED MIASM

This is the term used when a patient presents symptoms not only of an active miasm but also of the full symptom picture of the proven nosode of that miasm. *Psorinum* was made by Hahnemann from the infected discharge of a scabies vesicle, *Medorrhinum* is made from gonorrhoea pus, *Syphilinum* is made from an active syphilis product, and *Tuberculinum* from tuberculosis infected tissue. These nosodes have been given full provings and we have excellent pictures of them as remedies. *Carcinosin* is similarly a remedy made from cancer cells, this nosode has had only a limited proving, but there is a good picture of it built up from clinical experience which amounts to a clinical proving. When we see the clear picture of one of these nosodes we have an exposed miasm. There are many other nosodes and some have well known clinical indications in the materia medicas.

In Stanzas 206 – 209 Hahnemann instructs us to carefully individualise the case taking interview in order to see the symptoms which reflect the true needs of the patient. We cannot prescribe for a miasm which is not an individual quality. We prescribe a nosode, which is not the same as a miasm, when its known total symptom picture is clearly present.

ACUTE MIASM

Is the name given to infectious diseases which affect most people once in a lifetime, like measles and whooping cough, or diseases like yellow fever which are endemic to certain areas. In some individuals there are lasting ill-effects of these diseases and we may find an acquired miasm.

ARE MIASMS CONTAGIOUS?

Features of a dormant miasm cannot be transmitted or affect others except through inheritance. Symptoms of an active miasm can be transmitted and are contagious to those of a similar susceptibility. We can see that, for example, a previously healthy woman may develop a variety of urinary and reproductive problems as well as possibly other sycotic symptoms after a particular sexual relationship. This is a case of 'never been well since' the relationship, and occurs when the partner has an active sycotic miasm, most probably acquired from suppressed gonorrhoea.

An exposed miasm may have no 'active' aspects of the miasm and therefore may present no risk of contagion. However, an exposed miasm may also include some degree of active miasm and this would be contagious.

PRINCIPLE XII

Obstacles to cure depend on deep fundamental causes which are accurately described by the Theory of Miasms. These obstacles can be removed by correct homœopathic treatment.

Chapter 4 notes

EXAMPLES OF SOME MAJOR ANTI-MIASMATIC REMEDIES

PSORA *Sulphur, Calcarea Carbonica, Baryta Carbonica, Alumina, Graphites, Zincum, Petroleum, Carbo Animalis, Carbo Vegetalis, Mezereum, Sarsaparilla.*

SYCOSIS *Natrum Sulph, Pulsatilla, Sabina, Thuja, Cannabis Indica, Dulcamara, Lachesis.*

SYPHILIS *Aurum, Mercurius, Hepar Sulphuricum, Kali Iodatum, Platina, Palladium, Arsenicum, Phosphorous, Cocculus, Fluoric Acid, Kreosote, Manganum, Rhododendron, Rhus Toxicodendron, Stramonium, Nitric Acid.*

TUBERCULOSIS *Calcarea Phosphorica, Stannum, Rumex, Causticum, Drosera, Spongia, Silica.*

CANCER *Cadmium, Condurango, Hydrastis, Radium Bromide, Natrum Muriaticum, Staphysagria, Conium, Phytolacca.*

Some of these remedies are the great polychrest remedies which can cover the manifestations of all miasms and these lists are only an indication of the kind of picture the active miasm is capable of producing and are not exclusive.

CASE EXAMPLE

A case example to illustrate the cure of an active inherited miasm by the indicated remedy:

Boy. Date of birth 12/13/87. Case taken 12/10/90

His main presenting complaints centred around his behavioural problems which include obsessive ritualistic routines, eg won't go to sleep until every toy is in its place, he becomes upset by any change of plan. He finds difficulty receiving or displaying affection.

His family history includes cancer and his father had non-specific urethritis. There is tuberculosis on his mother's side. His birth was a difficult one; the labour went on for 14 hours and ended in a forceps delivery. He was in distress at birth; after the delivery he was very agitated and screamed for several hours. At the age of six weeks and again at three months he had the Diphtheria, Polio, Tetanus vaccination and at fifteen months received the vaccination against Measles, Mumps and Rubella; no specific bad reactions were noticed. In December 1988, he suffered from bronchitis which was treated with antibiotics.

His mother says he is basically a loving little boy who seems to be very worried about life. He is very imaginative, very sensitive and could be psychic. He is precocious in his play and vocabulary although socially backward. He is especially unaffectionate towards his father. He can be violent and jealous towards his younger sister. He has a bad temper, he contradicts and will hit his mother back if she smacks him. He still wears nappies, he cannot bear any change in his routine or anything to do with his body. He is afraid of water on his face and head. After his sister was born he would not sit down in the bath for six weeks. He is also afraid of the dark and can imagine faces coming out of the shadows. This fear has become more pronounced recently. He dislikes having his photograph taken and seems to be afraid of the flash. When he is hurt he runs away and will not let his mother touch him, any consolation makes him worse.

He loves music and dancing. Generally he sleeps well although often wakes at 4am. He complains that his bed is too hard. He usually goes to sleep lying on his abdomen.

He is a thirsty child and desires fruit, fruit juice, yogurt, cheese, bread and butter, crisps and salt. He can sometimes vomit if he eats oranges.

He gets hot easily and throws off his bed covers at night. He dislikes both the sun and heat. His head gets especially hot and sweaty. He enjoys bright, clear weather and hates wet weather and getting wet.

The prescriber who took the case could see symptoms which would partially indicate *Natrum Muriaticum, Aurum Metalicum, Sulphur, Stramonium* and *Medorrhinum.* However the case would not confirm or give an unequivocal clear picture of any of these remedies. Aetiological similarity was considered and Arnica and other birth trauma remedies were ruled out except for Natrum Sulph which fits the essence of the case. This is the main remedy for mental symptoms from injuries ("Synthetic Repertory" p20) and confirmed in Allen's "Keynotes and Characteristics". *Natrum Sulph* is one of the main remedies for aggravation from wet weather and wet, damp conditions (Kent's Repertory p1421) and again confirmed in Allen's "Keynotes". The general *Natrum* qualities of the child led to the overall picture being confirmed by the detailed materia medicas and the causation of inherited sycotic miasm, which came through the father's non-specific urethritis. A prescription of *Natrum Sulph 200* was given on 12/10/90.

First Report 16/10/90

There has been a great aggravation in the boy's behaviour, he has become more violent and aggressive. However he is sleeping better; previously he slept badly and disturbed his parent's sleep. He is also less afraid of the dark but he is more unhappy, depressed and capricious. The interpretation of this apparent aggravation on the higher levels was that the remedy had acted and we had to wait for the action to run its course before judging if this action was curative.

Second Report 2/11/90

There was a copious amount of green discharge from the nose and off the chest and this was followed by a cough which does not wake him. His behaviour has improved, he is a different child, pleasant, amenable and happy.

Third report 16/11/90

There has continued a night cough which does not wake him. He has become very imaginative, almost like a mature adult in his imagination and attitudes and continues improving psychologically.

EXERCISES

1. Read the picture of the main proven nosodes of *Psorinum*, *Medorrhinum* and *Syphilinum* in Tyler, Kent, and Clarke.
2. Define First Aid, Acute Disease and Chronic Disease. How do miasms relate to this scheme of the division of disease?
3. How does the theory of miasms relate to individual susceptibility?
4. Explain what is meant by a virus, bacterium or microbe and state whether you consider they cause disease in themselves.
5. How do you assess the impact of miasms on a patient?
6. How does the miasm theory help you improve diagnosis and prognosis of a patient?

RECOMMENDED READING FOR CHAPTER 4

Agarwal, YR 'A Comparative Study of Chronic Miasms'
Foubister, DM 'The Carcinosin Drug Picture' (IB & PS)
Hahneman, Samuel 'The Organon of Medicine', Stanzas 9-20
Hahneman, Samuel 'Chronic Diseases'
Kent, James Tyler 'Lectures on Homœopathic Philosophy',
    Chapters 3, 18-26
Roberts, Herbert 'The Principles, Art and Science of Homœopathy',
    Chapters 22-35
Vithoulkas, George 'The Science of Homœopathy', Chapters 8 and 9

Chapter V

WHAT IS TO BE CURED?

5.1 CAUSATION

This is an important idea in any study. At one extreme the cause of anything can be taken back to the original cause of all things – creation. At the other extreme, and the most common fallacy of modern times, is to look too shallowly at events. This brings about the famous 'regression fallacy', which is named after the statistical technique for showing the degree of association between two variables or post hoc ergo procter hoc (afterwards therefore because of). When one thing follows another you may say it is caused by that which precedes. However, if we look further we may see that both these things are in fact the result of yet another greater cause. For example, when statistics showed following the war, upward parallel trends in both the number of rape cases and attendances at church, this strong regression could not be taken as significant as both were responses to other larger causes in a changing society.

Similarly, the theories of causation that allopathic medicine offers are of a superficial nature since they do not embrace a theory of susceptibility which is sufficiently deep. Causative factors are sought in the blood, sputum, stool, urine and cerebro-spinal fluid alone, where investigators seek accompanying organisms to disease. These so called causes are however created by deeper causes. The changes in body chemistry and hormonal secretions are only a symptom and like the other symptoms of illness their true causes lie in the susceptibility of the patient. Homœopathic theory gives us an insight into the deeper, truer causes of disease. The theory of miasms is the cornerstone of this insight.

Causation or aetiology in homœopathy refers to a situation of 'never been well since'. In Kent's Repertory for example, we see rubrics beginning "Ailments From", these may be found in the Mind section under Fright and Grief. This indicates that the Vital Force was, in the normal course of time, unable to adapt fully to the trauma, and some ill effects remain which present as symptoms of importance. When a trauma has a profound effect on the patient, it adds a new layer, and this may have to be prescribed for before further progress can be made. The most common serious physical causes of such changes are vaccinations, modern medicinal drugs and surgery. Emotional traumas like rejection, fear, grief and humiliation and any strong emotion that is suppressed can also add a layer and require a 'never been well since' prescription. We prescribe this way, on a causation, either: i) when it dominates the case, or ii) when the seemingly well-chosen remedy fails to work and the aetiology in the case is strong. Sometimes this aetiological prescription acts to cure the patient, sometimes it does nothing discernible but after its use the remedy previously given to no avail now acts curatively.

5.2 VACCINATIONS

The vaccinations commonly given worldwide were never fully or properly tested before they were introduced on a mass scale. The literature given below gives growing evidence of the harmful effects of vaccination.

Vaccinations convert acute illnesses into long term chronic disease which is miasmatic in nature. There is mounting evidence of the ill effects of vaccination. The smallpox vaccination gives symptoms similar to the sycotic miasm or to symptoms generated after gonorrhoea has been suppressed. The polio vaccination sets up trouble in the brain, the central nervous system, the heart and the kidneys. There is a link between multiple sclerosis, meningitis and the polio vaccine.

Statistical evidence of the efficacy of vaccinations can easily be shown to be false. Vaccinations were introduced when the diseases in question were already on the decline due largely to improvements in sewerage and water supplies. Scarlet fever has no vaccine, yet it has declined exactly like the diseases that do have vaccinations. If an illness is reported and the patient has been vaccinated a different disease label (diagnosis) is often given; this produces false proof of the efficacy of the vaccination.

Vaccinations cause myriads of diseases from glue ear, dullness of mind, cot deaths, a failure of children to thrive and they also contribute to AIDS. Vaccinations deplete the immune system: when the vaccine is introduced directly into the blood stream the body's defence system has no time to build anti-bodies as it does have during the period of incubation afforded by the normal channels of infection, eg by droplet infection or sexual contact.

There is evidence that to delay the usual vaccinations in children reduces the severity of the poisoning, but as homœopathy offers safe and effective alternatives to conventional vaccinations no reason exists to continue the use of vaccination in the modern world. A gradual substitution of world wide vaccination programmes with good homœopathic clinics could be achieved within ten years.

5.3 DIAGNOSIS

To practice medicine we must know our patients, their environment, their culture, their family and social background. We must know what is normal in all these contexts and what is abnormal or pathological on all levels. Stanza 3 says it is necessary for the physicians to "...clearly perceive what is to be cured in diseases, that is to say, in every individual case of disease..."
Each disease will usually have two components:
1. The first consists of the common symptoms which are the more obvious parts of the Defence Posture.
2. The second group of symptoms are unusual ones which may seem strange, rare and peculiar. These will reflect the unique part of the individual's susceptibility and reaction to the disease. These are called characteristic symptoms or sometimes keynote symptoms.

The unenlightened physician relies on the first group of symptoms ignoring any peculiar ones and makes a diagnosis along the lines of a disease label which accommodates the commonly found symptoms. For example, ulcerative colitis or Addison's disease is diagnosed. Having made a diagnosis of this restrictive type the allopath hands over the function of cure to one of the commercial companies who manufacture drugs to make profit for their shareholders. In this way, physical symptoms which belong to the particular parts are normally given most, if not exclusive, importance. Any emotional or mental symptoms would be fitted into another disease label called 'mental disease' and the specialist in this area would try to fit the patient into one of the boxes called depression, schizophrenia or neurosis etc. This disease label approach to diagnosis reverses our preferred hierarchy in which most weight is given to 'individualising' symptoms which are the characteristic ones, followed in importance by mental and physical general symptoms and lastly by the common symptoms of the disease. (See Chapter 2)

The enlightened physician will make a diagnosis based on all levels which includes changes on the mental and emotional levels as well as physical changes and symptoms, thus obtaining a totality which is carefully graded into a hierarchy of importance and urgency and thus meet the patient's complete needs.

Concomitant symptoms are ones found in a system or organ or a level which is different from where the main complaint or disturbance lies. These concomittant disturbances often reflect the individual expression of the disease and can be characteristic, or strange, rare and peculiar. (See Diagram 8 in Chapter 3).

A diagnosis is an accurate assessment of the patient's complete needs. Diagnosis is the skill of seeing the true similarity between the image of the patient's symptoms and the image of a remedy. True similarity includes the totality of symptoms accurately graded according to intensity and urgency of impact on the patient now. Diagnosis is in fact an assessment of what is to be cured. To arrive at a complete homœopathic diagnosis we not only have to take the case, grade the symptoms, assess the importance of any aetiological factors and assess the depth and intensity of the physical symptoms, but we also often have to assess the effect of past and current drug use as many our patients will have been previously treated allopathically.

Laboratory tests may be useful in some cases but do not allow your patients to be exposed to invasive tests of any kind, these include those which tamper with the cerebro-spinal fluid. It is the duty of the homœopath to make a thorough examination of the patient on all levels. This may require a thorough clinical examination. It is necessary to seek further specialised help and advice when appropriate and the practitioner must know how to obtain such help which is safe and consistent with the highest ideals of the healing profession.

5.4 PROGNOSIS

Prognosis is the likely outcome of disease. A prognosis can be made, at least partially, after a full homœopathic diagnosis has been made. Prognosis depends on:

1. The clarity of the remedy picture. When a relatively healthy person becomes ill the Vital Force can show a clear picture of a homœopathic remedy. This indicates a good prognosis.
2. The centre of gravity of the case. If the pathology is very deep in the mental and emotional levels prognosis is less good.
3. The complexity of the case, a case with many layers will show a complexity of symptoms which will require long careful treatment. The prognosis might be less good in these cases but with careful prescribing and good cooperation from the patient the prognosis can be improved.
4. The seriousness or otherwise of the exciting cause. A serious decline in health which occurs from a slight cause like a change in diet or a slight chill or a minor disappointment indicates a seriously depleted immune system. The prognosis is less good.

So a poor prognosis may be the result of things like a history of deep and serious diseases, or traumas, or a lot of suppressive therapy including surgery or ECT treatment. Severe or prolonged drug abuse, including alcohol, also having had no childhood illnesses indicates a weak constitution.

PATIENTS' SENSITIVITY

If a patient is oversensitive there will be a poor prognosis. Oversensitivity can be guaged from the patient's reaction to past experiences. An extreme over-reaction shows pathological sensitivity just as an abnormal under-reaction indicates a poor vitality. Look for allergic reactions to medicine including other natural therapies, or vaccinations or to diets. There may be an over-reaction to world events and life circumstances. An intolerance of confrontation or critisism or an extreme over-concern with diet are also indications of oversensitivity

BLOCKAGES TO TREATMENT

George Vithoulkas describes four groups of people where the prognosis is poor because they block healing:

1. Spiritual seekers
2. Those with fixed ideas
3. Intellectuals
4. Those who fear becoming dependent on you and withdraw information and response.

5.5 WHAT IS TO BE CURED

The most difficult part of the art of homœopathic case management is deciding what it is you want to cure. Do you cure the disease lesion, which may be physical like eczema, sinusitis or thrush? Or do you cure strong mental symptoms like a fear of leaving the house or impulses to kill? Or do you cure not one thing but a syndrome or complex of symptoms?

We have described the dangers of removing or curing symptoms which are too superficial and which are the effects of deeper causes. We have described the wisdom of addressing our treatment to the Central Disturbance existing on the inner levels rather than directing our curative medicines at the peripheral or secondary symptoms (which, nevertheless, the patient often finds troublesome and consults us for the very purpose of having these 'peripheral' disturbances removed).

It will help to give a summary of what some of our teachers have said about this:

1. James Tyler Kent teaches us to treat the totality of the symptoms which are properly graded according to the hierarchy of importance.

2. George Vithoulkas, although flexibly adapting totality, keynote and essence to each case according to its needs, is best known for prescribing on the essence of the case. The essence is very close to the concept of the 'Central Disturbance', a term popularised by Dr Rajan Sankaran.

3. A third emphasis says that the Central Disturbance is often shown best by the mental generals, confirmed and supported by the physical generals. Many homœopaths seek to "generalise the particulars", which is a way of seeing the impress of the individual patient's inner nature on the disease pathology. For example, when the anxiety, the pains and the organic dysfunction appear only between 4.00pm to 8.00pm we can say there is a general symptom of a 4 to 8pm aggravation and use this symptom as more important than the particular anxiety, pains and difficulty.

4. Thomas Maughan taught that the 'needs' of the patient were to be met, and curative remedies based on similarity, were to be aimed at meeting these true needs. This would not necessarily be what the patient presented to you to cure, it also has to be carefully distinguished from what you, the prescriber, may want. Often the prescriber's interpretations of the patient's symptoms and needs are coloured by the their own prejudices. Here are a few examples:

"If I clear up this disease it will prove to the rest of the medical profession how good I am."

"If I give this patient what he wants he will approve of me and I value the prestige of this."

"This person needs to fit in with one of my belief systems so what they are really trying to say is... and I shall prescribe accordingly."

"I am afraid of this pathology and possible consequences of treating it so I will palliate this case and pass it on."

To meet the patient's inner and complete needs is difficult. We have to:
1. Take the case in a detached manner.
2. Assess the totality, essence, keynotes and causations of the case.
3. See what is the correct grading of symptoms. This is the process whereby we decide on the 'true needs' of the patient.

The word hierarchy relates the patient's symptoms to a model of correct hierarchical order. This must be consistent with the reality of universal hierarchy. (See Chapter 1)

5.6 CASE ANALYSIS PART 1 – TYPES OF CASES

Stanza 3 poses the question of whether the physician sees what is to be cured. It is fruitless deciding what is to be cured a priori, each patient presents a unique case and only when we understand the individual nature of that case can we decide on what is to be cured.

If the case itself is correctly taken and correctly analysed that will tell us clearly what is to be cured. Case analysis means making a correct assessment of the important features of the case and discovering the centre of gravity or the mainspring of all the symptoms which motivates and creates the individual and their world.

Each individual case will look quite different, we may find:

1. Patients who have serious physical pathology involving tissue change like, eczema, psoriasis, ulcerative colitis, angina, pericarditis, multiple sclerosis or cancer.
2. Patients who have a poorly functioning organ or system like the kidneys, bladder, liver or a ductless gland, a poor circulation or rheumatic pains.
3. Diseases of the sensory organs like Meniere's Disease, which is characterised by tinnitus, deafness and intermittent attacks of dizziness possibly accompanied by nausea and sweating.
4. Patients may present with serious psychological problems like, insomnia, fears, anxieties, depression or phobias. Patients with these more serious problems may have only relatively minor physical problems.
5. Patients with diagnosed mental states like schizophrenia, manic depression or advanced phobias of one kind or another. This group is distinguished from group four by the deeper penetration or longer standing of the disease and also because they would usually also belong to the next class of patients.

6.   Patients who are taking conventional medicines which are neither super-ficial or very recent.

7.   Patients who present with acute pain and seek immediate relief. This may be a fresh episode or a recurrence of a chronic condition which has been quiescent for a while. This may include headaches, gall or kidney colics, neuralgias, gout etc.

8.   We may occasionally find patients who enjoy perfect health except for one condition, eg bed wetting in children or an isolated pain or acne.

The decision of where to aim your remedy prescription, your decision about what is to be cured, now has to be made. You must always take into account the patient's wishes, although the patient's views must not be allowed to override your professional knowledge and judgement. This is a difficult balance to maintain especially with patients who are demanding and forceful in pursuit of what they want. This moment of assessment before making your prescription choice and after taking the case to the best of your abilities is a time fraught with dangers. This is a time when your own preju-dices can influence the course of events, or when your interaction with the patient can spoil your detachment. Before continuing with this crucially important case assessment and analysis process I would like to consider some differing approaches to case analysis.

5.7 DIFFERENT APPROACHES OF CASE ANALYSIS

Different practitioners hold in their minds different models and seek to see each case in the light of that model and how this model opens up the case to reveal a remedy picture. The range of models varies from those requiring great openness of mind and flexibility to those at the other extreme which force the patients individuality into a fixed mould.

Diagram 8 shows this range.

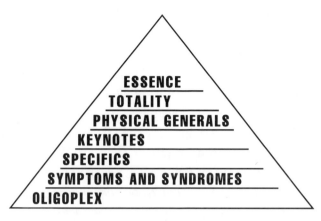

Diagram 8

1. **The Essence**. This is the mainspring of the individual, it reflects a deep rooted posture expressed mainly by the subconscious in dreams, delusions and fears, but often also given to the carefully observing physician by gestures, repeated phrases and themes, or in unguarded statements or confidences.

2. The essence should be supported by **The Totality of Symptoms** properly graded. This carefully valued totality can often guide you to the essence.

3. **Physical Generals.** If an essence is recalcitrant in showing itself and the totality seems diffused a careful look at the physical generals, including temperature reaction, perspiration, food desires, sleep pattern, reaction to pressure, touch, motion, weather, locality and the time of day etc may give an indication of the remedy. Also if we can determine the general qualities of the particular symptoms and this conforms to the overall pattern, a clear picture may be seen. The physical generals are important with patients who show a confused mental picture with few or conflicting keynotes or with so many varied mental symptoms it is hard to see a single remedy picture in them.

4. **Keynotes** are spectacular symptoms. They are characteristic of the patient; things which are said to be typical of the patient like strange rare

and peculiar symptoms which are strong. Most times we prescribe on keynotes in first aid, and acutes which demand urgent attention or when there is an acute or sub-acute condition giving a top layer of urgent need. Sometimes this will be a minor remedy not as frequently indicated as the first-aid remedies or the polycrests and major nosodes. Sometimes in complex many-layered cases a keynote prescription of a relatively minor remedy will open the case by dealing with the top layer. Be careful not to prescribe on one or even two keynotes, these may often be aberrant symptoms from another layer. The old school taught to have a "three legged stool and one other," ie four keynotes.

5. **Specifics** refers to the use of specific remedies for disease labels eg *Cantharis* for cystitis, *Drosera* for whooping cough, *Lachesis* for hot flushes. This technique ignores the first principle of healing, that of individualisation. Any remedy can have any disease, it is our duty to carefully individualise each case from first-aid and acute illnesses to chronic conditions. In every case we proceed according to the scheme laid out in Diagram 8, which gives the areas that you have to explore in order to find all the symptoms of the situation, these are sensation, location, extension, modalities, causation and concomittants. The specifics approach to treating every case is not to be confused with 'therapeutics' which is a study of the details of remedies so as to differentiate them in cases where the physical symptoms or particulars need careful and urgent treatment thus finding the most similar remedy to the patient's uppermost needs at the time.

6. **Symptoms and Syndromes** This refers to the practice of treating symptoms or groups of symptoms regardless of the needs of the patient as a whole. This was discussed under 'suppression' in Chapter 2.

7. **Oligoplex** follows inevitably from suppression – why take any chances? Give the patient several remedies known to be 'homœopathic' to the condition they complain of; so several remedies are given at one time and also repeated frequently.

5.8 THE ORIGIN OF DIFFERENT TYPES OF SYMPTOM PICTURES OF DISEASE

We can divide symptoms according to quantity and quality. The quantity of symptoms will depend on the strength of the Vital Force. When the disease in the central state requires some form of outward expression it will do this in the least harmful way possible. The vitality will govern the quantity of symptoms. What governs the quality of these symptoms? It is the constitution, which in turn depends on the diatheses or miasmatic influences. This gives us four possibilities as to the types of cases we will find:

Group I The vitality is good and the constitution is strong; this will give us plenty of symptoms of a good quality so they form a clear picture of a homœopathic remedy.

Group II The vitality is poor so there are few symptoms but the constitution is good so the quality of the symptoms is good. Few symptoms but of good quality would give us keynotes of one remedy so a good prescription is possible.

Group III In this group there is a good vitality which gives us plenty of symptoms but the constitution is poor having been weakened by many miasmatic influences so that the quality of symptoms is poor. In this group we find those cases which seem to have many layers of disease. From each layer comes a few symptoms. The total effect is many symptoms but not one remedy picture, there will be a confusing and conflicting array of symptoms.

Group IV Here the vitality is low and the constitution is poor. We have few symptoms of a poor quality. If there are any keynotes or characteristic symptoms they will be isolated or conflicting. The few symptoms present do not fit into any one clear remedy picture. These are the cases of broken down constitutions, with an accretion of acquired miasms and a debilitated Vital Force. Into this group would come incurable cases, also those cases which have many layers and where many of the constitutional and general symptoms have faded away before a more serious pathology either physical or mental.

It is the complex cases found in groups III and IV which give us most difficulty. Deciding what is to be cured can sometimes be difficult in these cases.

When we take the case properly and review the patient's whole life biography, together with their inheritance we are able to assess what is important in the case.

To decide what is to be cured we should consider:

- Any urgent or intense symptoms which may threaten danger to life or cause further serious pathology if neglected.
- An analysis of what is innermost or causative which includes any dominant similarity like aetiology which shapes the whole case.
- An analysis of the layers and their location and a decision as to which layer has to be treated first.

Before we go onto detailed analysis of layered cases let us remind ourselves of the aims of homœopathy. These include:

1. To cure the disease which troubles the patient by finding its true cause and removing it, but furthermore
2. To build health and to strengthen both vitality and constitution so that there is no relapse into the previous diseased state again. To do both these things you must see the true needs of the patient, which is seeing what the patient needs to do in order to make their next step in their conscious development to fulfil their purpose in life.
3. The third purpose of homœopathic prescribing is controversial and can be described as assisting the patient along their evolutionary path.

5.9 BEFORE THE FIRST PRESCRIPTION

When you see a patient your first assessment must be of the urgency of the needs of the patient. Is it a first-aid situation or the kind of acute manifestation that requires immediate attention? Is the case a long term chronic one and if so what is its nature? The steps you take are to carefully receive the accurate and unprejudiced symptom totality including:

- A diligent inquiry into the inheritance.
- A clear chronology from conception to the present time.

- A note of any aetiological similarities where past events are still affecting the patient.

You then grade all of these symptoms and elements into a correct hierarchy of importance.

In this case-taking and assessment process you will probably have used the repertories to look at key rubrics and finally you will consult the materia medicas to identify the correct remedy for the patient. However, before deciding on the first prescription the following additional steps are recommended:

- Pause, look at the patient and see if the remedy you have chosen suits the real person sitting before you.
- Discuss with the patient any possible maintaining causes, likely antidotes and other possible hindrances to health which are present. These may include suitable diet, life-style, use of pleasure or prescribed drugs, use of the contraceptive pill, social and work relationships or living difficulties. All of these issues should be discussed with the patient as an equal. Offer your knowledge and advice only insofar as the issue affects the efficacy of your prescription and treatment. This whole case assessment process puts into perspective the patient's whole life needs, the role of the prescription you are about to give and also further informs you of the appropriateness of your remedy choice and what it can hope to achieve (prognosis).

THE WORK OF A HOMŒOPATH COVERS THREE ASPECTS

1. To prescribe correctly according to the needs of the patient shown by the correctly graded symptoms.
2. To educate patients about the true nature of healing, the role of the healer and the responsibilities of the patient.
3. To advise patients when they ask for advice. When patients come to see you they are open to some degree of change in their lives. You should advise honestly according to your own knowledge and training, but often patients will need advice from someone skilled in other techniques, such as counselling. You should be able to advise them as to the form of fur-

ther help and advice they may need and know who to recommend in other disciplines. Some examples of other skills you may recommend are included in the Notes to this Chapter.

You must always be aware of the possibility that the patient may not at this moment require a medicine. There may be other things which need to be done first. In Stanza 225 Hahnemann discusses this possibility and concludes that in some patients

> *It is only such emotional diseases as these, which were first engendered and subsequently kept up by the mind itself, that, while they are yet recent and before they have made any great inroads on the corporeal state, may, by means of psychical remedies, such as a display of confidence, friendly exhortations, sensible advice, and often by a well-disguised deception, be rapidly changed into a healthy state of the mind (and with appropriate diet and regimen, seemingly into a healthy state of the body also).*
>
> *Stanza 226*

Similarly we occasionally see patients who are already seeing a counsellor or other therapist. It may be that the other healing produces favourable changes and progress. You should not further interfere by prescribing. Note all the changes and symptoms on each level and wait until there is a need for a further stimulation when a homœopathic prescription can help the patient take the next step.

There is a distinction between therapies that can work side by side with homœopathic treatment and those which would be disruptive to take at the same time. (See Notes)

Chapter 5 notes

CASE EXAMPLE

A case example where the common disease symptoms give a diagnosis but taking the patient's individual symptoms led to the curative remedy.

Case No.AC17 – College Clinic.

Baby girl. LR. Date of Birth 21/6/90. Case taken 4/10/90.

The baby's main presenting complaint was diagnosed as infantile colic. She has great pain and much wind with the colic. She screams with the pains. When she has the pain she draws her knees up onto her chest. The baby was obviously in great distress with the pains.

The colic began when she was 3 months old; no causative factors could be found.

The pregnancy and birth were normal although she was born 6 weeks prematurely. She was fed naso-gastrically 3 or 4 times while in hospital. She is now feeding 2 hourly and seems to be thriving well. She has had no vaccinations.

She prefers to sleep on her abdomen and her neck sweats when she is asleep.

She is also suffering from nappy rash which appears to be very red and sore.

A remedy, *Colocynthus,* was chosen on the basis of the severe abdominal pains which were improved by drawing her knees up.

Three days later:

No real improvement.

The mother noticed that she seemed a little better if she could expel some of the wind by burping; and also that the pains were worse between 5 and 8pm.

The baby enjoys cool breezes.

She has a little diarrhoea with a green-coloured stool.

On the diagnosis of trapped wind two remedies were selected which were well-indicated. *Carbo Vegetalis* gave a little improvement, but *Lycopodium* caused no change.

Three days later:

No change in her condition.

She may either bend double by drawing her knees up or stretch out during the pains. The pains make her very cross, irritable and difficult to please.

On these symptoms the remedy *Chamomilla* was chosen.

Three days later:

Baby arrived at the Acute Clinic with diarrhoea. The stool is yellow and loose. She is still suffering from much wind and abdominal pain.

Two more remedies with a reputation for curing infantile colic were selected, *Borax* and *Aethusa.*

One week later:

Baby still in great distress with the colic and the wind. No change after the previous remedies.

The mother noticed that the baby weeps in her sleep.

Ignoring the diagnosis with its common symptoms a remedy was chosen on the individual symptoms of the baby; ie a great improvement on being in fresh air, a great improvement while in her pram, ie during motion, and a strong dislike of being indoors. The remedy chosen was *Pulsatilla* which relieved all the abdominal symptoms and cured the case.

This case illustrates that the diagnosis is not all important and can get in the way of finding the curative remedy. The remedies chosen on the diagnoses of infantile colic and trapped wind did not improve the baby's condition. Only when the important symptoms of the case were taken and analysed did the correct remedy emerge.

ALTERNATIVE METHODS OF DIAGNOSIS

Alternative methods of obtaining diagnostic information so as to avoid invasive conventional diagnostic tests.

REFLEXOLOGY
Reflexology is an ancient healing art which uses a specific form of massage applied to the feet. Many conditions can be detected through the feet; reflexologists consider the feet to be a mirror of the body, reflecting the tensions and diseases which may be present.

SPINAL TOUCH THERAPY
By observing the spine and its deviations from a straight plum line, various internal disorders can be ascertained. Imbalance of the body or posture distortion usually indicates internal body changes long before any body functions appear disturbed. Any posture shift changes the position of all the organs placing them under strain and if this strain continues it can lead to disease. Light touch techniques on key areas of the spine redirect the inner energies of the body, allowing muscles to relax and gently re-establish the spine into its natural position aligned with gravity.

CRANIAL SACRAL THERAPY
Compression of the cranial bones and membranes by an accident or birth trauma can impair normal development of the brain and many problems can arise. Cranial sacral therapy works to restore balance to the bones and membranes of the cranium so that the brain can grow and develop normally.

IRIDOLOGY OR IRIS DIAGNOSIS

Every part of the body relates to a section of the iris. By studying the iris problems and imbalances can be pinpointed. Illnesses past and present can still be visible, recorded in the iris pattern as dark spots over the organ area, and nutritional imbalances affect the iris colour.

PSYCHIC HEALERS

Psychic healers of known qualities are able to give a medical diagnosis out of their work.

CHAKRA ANALYSIS

The Chakras (wheels) are the centres of energy at seven key points along the spinal column. Those skilled in this technique are able to gauge the strength and quality of the energy flow in each Chakra and diagnose areas of disease from their knowledge of what each Chakra represents on all levels of the human economy.

CHINESE/JAPANESE DIAGNOSIS

This refers to the Eastern art of making diagnoses about internal states and organs by observing the colour, shape and texture of external parts, notably the face and tongue.

APPLIED KINESIOLOGY

This considers the relationships of muscles to internal organs and the acu-pressure energy that passes through them, thus connecting them dynami-cally. Allergy testing using Applied Kinesiology, observes the fact that a muscle will test weak in the presence of an allergen. The body instinctively knows the foods to which it is sensitive; the vitamins and minerals it is lack-ing etc.

THERAPIES COMPLEMENTARY TO HOMŒOPATHY

If a form of therapy is effective, conforms to the correct direction of cure, follows the principles of wholism – individual healing and minimal interference – then it is consistent with the highest ideals of healing. Two such therapies should not be received by a patient at the same time and there has to be a choice as to whether homœopathy or another therapy should be received. To have both treatments at the same time would be the equivalent of giving two major remedies at the same time and we would lose control of the case. However some therapies can work with homœopathic treatment at the right time and in full co-operation with the prescribing homœopath. Some examples might be:

1   Constructive counselling
2   Metamorphic technique
3   Sacro spinal therapy
4   Healing – spiritual or psychic
5   Co-counselling
6   Alexander lessons
7   Spinal touch therapy
8   Cranial osteopathy
9   Yoga which includes all the Eight limbs of Yoga
10 Crystal healing

THERAPIES CONFLICTING WITH HOMŒOPATHY

Those therapies that would conflict with ongoing homœopathic treatment and are advisable to take only when homœopathic treatment is finished (unless used only for diagnosis) include:

1   Acupuncture
2   Reflexology
3   Bach Flower Remedies
4   Healing

5   Shiatsu massage
6   Vitamin therapy
7   Dietary therapy
8   Hypnotherapy

FACTORS AFFECTING PROGNOSIS

Factors which affect the response to the homœopathic interview and treatment which are important for prognosis are:

1. The most important is the will to live. One aspect of this is seen in the will to health, the presence of which can work wonders. The other aspect of this is in the will to escape pain or discomfort. Patients motivated only by the desire to escape pain are more difficult patients for the homœopath to deal with since there may be an exacerbation of suffering on the way to the state of health and they will not like/tolerate this or easily change the contributing habits. Patients motivated by the desire to improve their health and are willing to change the maintaining causes are the most easy to work with and are usually quite able to understand the apparent ups and downs of homœopathic treatment.

2. Ability to live a happy life, (ability to adjust to the misfortunes of life; a capacity for joy, wonder; an appreciation of beauty and of nature). Remember that dis-ease is produced by inability to adjust to changes – at whatever level of our being.

3. Their image of themselves (the 'miserable sinner' who tells himself that he has no health in him will, of course, have no health in him). The self-image is a powerful limiter of expression. Much research has taken place into this idea in the field of psychology, creative realisation, Science of Mind, etc This is one of the areas in which the prescriber must also be a teacher, if he is to be a healer.

4. The limit of their horizons (the 'what I know is what is true/real/all that needs to be known. Everything which differs is lies/false/useless/nonsense/superstition/unscientific, etc). The definition of this criteria

depends on the horizons of the Homœopath. Fixed ideas for small minds or, 'the world's your oyster'.

5. If they have protected themselves from stress (needlessly dependent on Social Security or hospital, churches, drugs, alcohol, or habitually uses Valium, or uses less obvious ways of self protection). This means a much reduced ability to adjust to changes.

6. If they have isolated themselves from relationships with others or changed partners very frequently this shows again an overprotection process.

7. Ability to make human contact with the homœopath. Some patients will have a freedom in their relationships and some will be very tightly closed. Some 'flow' and others will be toxic with 'stagnation'.

CHAPTER V EXERCISES

1. Define diagnosis giving all the elements required for a complete homœopathic diagnosis, where does the usual allopathic diagnosis fit into this?
2. Define prognosis. What are the main areas of information which determine the prognosis both before and after the first prescription?
3. In patients with a poor vitality there will be few symptoms. What is it that weakens vitality?
4. Are the concepts of vitality and constitution, which were discussed in Section 8, easily related or interconnected?
5. Is a broken down constitution the same as a weakened vitality?
6. Relate the concepts of susceptibility to the arguments in favour of vaccination and those against vaccination, eg if you have a susceptibility to a particular disease will the vaccination be harmful, necessary or beneficial?
7. In your own words explain how causation can be both too superficial and too profound to be valuable in homœopathic case taking. What is the correct perception and use of causation?

RECOMMENDED READING FOR CHAPTER V

Burnett, J Crompton 'Vaccinosis, and its cure by Thuja' World Homœopathic
    Links, New Delhi

Chaitow, Leon 'Vaccination and Immunisation' C W Daniel, Revised 1991

Clarke, J H 'Clinical Repertory' Part II, Health Science Press

Coulter, Harris 'DPT A Shot in the Dark' North Atlantic Books, California

Hahnemann, Samuel 'The Organon of Medicine' Stanzas 3, 71-90, 108,
    148-192, 205-207, Indian Books and Periodicals Syndicate

Hahnemann, Samuel 'Chronic Diseases' Jain

James, Walene 'Immunization: The Reality Behind the Myth' Bergin and
    Garvey 1988

Kent, James Tyler 'Lectures on Homœopathic Philosophy'
    Chapters 3, 17, 22, 23, 24, 25,m 26, 27, 35, Set Day & Co

Moskowitz, R 'The Case Against Immunizations' Homœopath 1984 4(4) 114-
    41 (available from SOH office)

Neustaedter, Randall 'The Immunization: A Guide for Parents' North Atlantic
    Books 1990

Neustaedter, Randall 'Measles and Homœopathic Vaccinations'
    Homœopath 1990 10(z) 31-32, 42

Nossaman, N J 'More about Immunizations' Journal of American Institute of
    Homœopathy 1983 9 89-99

Roberts, Herbert 'The Principles, Art and Practice of Homœopathy' Chapters
    9, 10, 11, Jain

Sankaran, D P 'The Importance of Aetiology in Homœopathy – A
    Symposium' The Homœopathic Medical Publishers

Shepherd, Dorothy 'Epidemic Diseases' Health Science Press

Vithoulkas, George 'The Science of Homœopathy'
    Chapters 9, 12, 13, 14, ASOHM 1978

Wright Hubbard, Elizabeth 'A Brief Study Course in Homœopathy'
    Chapters 11, 12, I B & P S

INDEX